STRONGHOLDS OF THE MIND

Biblical Remedies for Addictions

By

ALEXANDER GYIMAH AGYEMANG

DISCIPLESHIP SERIES

COPYRIGHT PAGE

Strongholds Of The Mind: Biblical Remedies For Addictions

© Alexander Gyimah Agyemang

First Published in March, 2020

ENLIGHTENED WORD TEACHING MINISTRY

C/O Post, Office Box 783, Takoradi Western Region, Ghana / West Africa

E-mail: lexgyi@yahoo.com **or** lexgyi@gmail.com

Lexgyi.blogspot.com

Instagram: lexgyi

Facebook.com / lexgyi@yahoo.com

Youtube: Alexander Gyimah Agyemang

Twitter.com/LEXGYI

Published by Amazon.com,USA

DEDICATION

I dedicate this Holy Spirit Inspired Book to my one and only sweetheart Mrs. Irene Gyimah Agyemang who has been my greatest cheerleader, believing in my anointing and gifts more than I sometimes believe myself. And To All Who By the Grace of God Have Overcome on Addiction which Use To Control Their Lives.

PREFACE

The world is plagued by people who are addicted to one thing or the other. People whose addictions are ruining families, causing deaths and generally leading many away from Godly counsel. Many blamed their inability to make meaningful impact in life on spiritual forces and enemies whilst neglecting to mention the skeletons in their closet, addictions which took most of their focus. Many people have had repeated prayers for progress in life to no avail because they failed to deal with the chief enemy within, their addictions.

This book has been written because there is a gap in knowledge when it comes to addiction, amongst the churches in the developing world. So much has been written on demons and witches but not on addictions amongst Christians and the biblical ways to deal with it. This book therefore contains comprehensive information on addictions and the havoc they are causing all over the world. This book even uncovers some addictions that most people are unaware of and explains why knowledge on them is important for a comprehensive fight against it.

This book prescribes ways of dealing with addictions which control the spirit, mind and body. It has also prescribed Biblical methods for treating addictions which deal with behavioural, emotional, substance and desire based addictions. These solutions are comprehensive and more effective than many therapies in use today which give the addicts substitute substances instead of the addictive one. Remembers which in itself can also create another dependency if used for too long.

I have shared my experiences as I battled with addictions as a young man growing up and have also drawn from the many former addicts who are now serving God as founders of churches, pastors, lay ministers and even businessmen and women. Read this book prayerfully and the lessons in it will transform your life and the lives of people around you battling addictions of all sorts.

Addictions need to be dealt with because they are the number one reason, Christians become hypocrites. Because Christians are ashamed of their addictions, they hide them. If the addictions are sinful then they act righteous to the outside world whilst secretly practising this sin. Thank God! The Bible has remedies for this canker.

The Author

TABLE OF CONTENTS   **PAGE**

SECTION 1: ADDICTION AS A STRONGHOLD OF THE MIND

CHAPTER 1

STRONGHOLDS OF THE MIND

Introduction

Every baby is adorable, why? Because they are curious in their own way and find interesting ways to communicate as much as can be understood by parents and guardians. The baby then grows to a helpless infant who starts to crawl, knocking things all over the place. At this stage their 'coolness' begins to reduce because their curiosity begins to upset the status quo in their parents or guardians house.

As this once adorable baby grows in adventure and begins to cause breakages and many messy situations in the home front. Parents and guardians start seeing him or her as a burden. At this stage 'baby adorable' begins to acquire new names like baby troublesome or baby messy. Then baby toddler starts to walk and things get even untidier. All things important and dangerous will then have to be kept from their reach if daddy and mommy want their peace of mind.

A lot of these naughty behaviours stops once baby toddler becomes a young child and can understand the basic do's and don'ts in the family and society at large. Even here, many children still do things which upset their parents, especially when they act in a group. The boys especially become even more adventurous as they try to prove to their peers and seniors that they are strong and likeable. As children become adolescent and even teens this sense of adventure increases in others whilst those with healthy family relationships at home rather tend to bond with family the more.

Girls and boys with less desirable relationships at home tend to seek it outside amongst friends and class mates. The tendency to pick the habits of this peer group because he or she wants to belong is almost certain. The habits which lead to addictions are some of those habits young people pick to show friends they are tough, adventurous or that they can be trusted to keep secrets of the group.

Habits

Habits are repeated behaviours or tendencies which have formed from years of repeated actions. Habits are usually things we do without conscious thoughts guiding it. Habits are the body's autopilot mechanism which it uses to free the brain from guiding all the millions of things we do as humans in a day, especially at the cellular level where a lot of processes are happening in our bodies.

The brain turn to record actions that it has learnt to repeat over several trials on reflex so it can concentrate on newer tasks that it is not familiar with. Habit therefore, are the actions that the body or mind takes that the brains is so familiar with that they have been put on auto pilot mode to happen when the preconditions are right.

There was a senior in my secondary school who was a genius when it came to answering science questions. My school being one of the best schools in Ghana was very competitive when it came to order of merit. But this senior of mine could top the entire science class for a number of terms consistently. A very unusual thing to be achieved for even the brightest in the school.

This senior was so good at answering questions that he could bow his head doing something else in class and just lift his head up in the middle of a calculation by a teacher and spot an error that the rest of his mates watching the board intently could not see. Because of this habit of excellence people will wait till he was asleep because he was a very busy student and then wake him up in the middle of his sleep to ask him to solve questions they were having difficulties with.

He will get up from bed sit down and give an excellent explanation whilst solving the question. After he had finished he will then go back to bed: most of the time after he woke up from bed in the morning he had no recollection of the entire episode. It appeared he tackled the questions whilst not fully conscious. His brain had recorded his constant tackling of questions of that nature and had put it on autopilot.

This tendency of the brain to automate many things that we do repeatedly is what leads to habits, character traits and addictions. Forming a new habit according to James Clear, 2018 takes more than 2 months

On average, it takes more than 2 months before a new behaviour becomes automatic — 66 days to be exact. And how long it takes a new habit to form can vary widely depending on the behaviour, the person, and the circumstances. In Lally's study, it took

anywhere from 18 days to 254 days for people to form a new habit. In other words, if you want to set your expectations appropriately, the truth is that it will probably take you anywhere from two months to eight months to build a new behaviour into your life — not 21 days. Interestingly, the researchers also found that "missing one opportunity to perform the behaviour did not materially affect the habit formation process." In other words, it doesn't matter if you mess up every now and then. Building better habits is not an all-or-nothing process.

Character

Character is essentially habits you are addicted to, behaviours or tendencies which have suited you so well that you have assumed them and internalised them. Character is a product of the interaction between yourself and the environment. Character is a set of reactions you have demonstrated so often that the brain has set them on auto pilot whenever similar situations arise.

Humans are ultimately the product of their environment. Because subconsciously, we are all aware that character is not cast in stone. Many people when life demands, they change a character flaw or seek for external help to overcome that weakness.

Many people need motivation whether good or bad to make quick changes to their character. Character result from years of programming which can be altered with the right influences or support. I believe no man is constantly within the character he is known for 24hrs of the day. A proof of what I am saying are the shocking things people we have known for decades do that we never thought they were capable of. Character is not a set behaviour but the average behaviour traits of an individual.

Mind

Romans 8:5-6 King James Version (KJV)

5 For they that are after the flesh do mind the things of the flesh; but they that are after the Spirit the things of the Spirit. 6 For to be carnally minded is death; but to be spiritually minded is life and peace.

From the scripture above the mind is what captures out attention as human beings. What you pay attention to is what is on your mind. What you think about all the time is something which has occupied your mind. What you think about all the time becomes a self-fulfilling prophecy concerning you. Job walked about with fear that all he had built could crumble and lo it happened to him on one fateful day. Concentrating only on things which please the flesh will make you weak in the spirit and expose you to the attacks of the devil. But if your mind is centred on spiritual things you will become more spiritual and therefore stronger to face the devil and his schemes.

What is the mind then? *The mind is a set of cognitive faculties including consciousness, perception, thinking, judgement, language and memory. It is usually defined as the faculty of an entity's thoughts and consciousness.*

The mind simply put, is the part of you which gives you your personality, your attitudes, habits, intelligence, languages, memory and self-awareness. Some people call it the soul or the part of you which defines your personality. The brain controls all the conscious functions the human being undertakes and ensures that the right environment has been created for the automatic processes happening in the body. The body is undergoing millions of processes simultaneously all the time at the cellular or organic levels without conscious instructions from the brain.

The brain has sections which control speech, consciousness, memory, judgement, perception, language yet the brain and mind are not the same. Why? Because people lose consciousness during accidents or during major surgical operations.

But are still able to perform these functions in another state of consciousness in a near death experience. They are able to see, remember, judge, speak and even observe themselves in the accidents scene or in the theatre without the support of their brain which might be comatose at the time. The mind is important because it controls our decisions especially our beliefs, perceptions, tendencies and ultimately our personalities. These are the very things which get altered or hijacked during addictions.

It is like a computer virus taking control of the computer's controlling system by altering the source code of the operating system. The virus then becomes the primary code that is running the system. A situation which is normally referred to as the 'hacking of a system'. In situations like that, you will need someone with the virus's source code to be able to remove it from the system and reinstate the old program. A similar method is employed to deal with addictions.

Stronghold

According to the Merriam Webster Dictionary a *stronghold is a fortified place, a place of security or survival, a place dominated by a particular group or marked by a particular characteristic.*[3] A stronghold essentially keeps what is within it from foreign invasion, it maintains the dominant characteristics of the place it is meant to protect. Strongholds built for trading in ancient times or for military purposes where fortified or structured to be impenetrable and had greater ammunitions outside of it to defend it against invaders. Mostly they were built at difficult places to attack like a hill or it was surrounded by a river to even make it more difficult to attack. There are many forts and castles dotted on the coast of West Africa which were used as strongholds for the trans-Atlantic slave trade..

They were so well built that most have survived without much maintenance for over two centuries. Most of them are the only surviving building in the area built more than two centuries ago. A testament to the strength of strongholds: even without active maintenance in difficult environments like the beaches they are still standing from sometimes as far as the eighteenth century.

My visit to the Cape coast and Elmina castles

These castles where built with a very difficult entrance. One had to wait for a draw bridge to be lowered down before you can enter. The bridge could only be operated by the guards at the gate. The gate had been designed such that it could only be operated when the main gates were opened. The bridge is over a man-made canal with deep waters within it, falling into that canal with the heavy armour of the time was certain death.

Because it was nearly impossible to climb out of those steep walls.

When we entered the castles we notice that it was seated on a hill overlooking the ocean. Standing in the castles gave you a view of miles upon miles of the ocean: a strategic point to see enemies miles ahead before they could get close enough to shoot their cannon balls at the castle. Facing the ocean were pointed several canons with cannon balls to shoot at the approaching enemy. The castle were built to be self-contain: there were dungeons, chapels, halls, armoury, places for building weapons, and even a grave yard.

To even secure themselves further they made friends with the local people where the castle was situated and released children they had with the slaves into the environment to stay around them. The trade in slaves became the main stay of these castles and the huge profit made in the trade attracted many European nations to Cape Coast. Typical of most strongholds the darkest secret it kept was buried deep within, in dungeons below with capacity to hold thousands of this human cargo.

This need to create wealth became an addiction to the slave traders resulting in them reducing fellow human beings to mere cargo. On top of this horror going on in the dungeons was their chapel, their suppose conscience as Christian nations at the time. From these castles or forts the Europeans ruled the vast expanse of Ghana like other West African countries for over a century. A testimony of the power of strongholds to empower the few to rule over the majority.

Strongholds of the mind

The mind as has been explained earlier is our personality, the control centre as far as our decisions and emotions are concern. The filter of our tendencies at it draws from decisions favoured by our character or temperament. The things we do by reason of habits, culture or training. Strongholds of the mind are therefore emotions, habits, or tendencies which have been fortified in our minds.

Things we do because they are our culture or because it reinforces our personalities. Things we do because they have served as well over the years. Things we do because of the level of our spiritual maturity. Things which have become our nature, culture or way of life. Acts which defined us or identify as individuals or as a collective.

Attitudes which are not helping us but we are heavily promoting because they are fortified in our minds under the tradition and culture we subscribe to. Things we do even when resident in developed countries where they are frown upon. Habits we will repeat even when we are staying with the pope or with the president of the United States of America. Things we do by default: things we do without reason or without recourse to the inspired word of God that we claim to live by.

I love Garri

Most Ghanaians who were boarders in secondary schools love Garri. Garri is dried cassava, a kind of cassava flakes. It was when I travelled to the UK where I had to eat cornflakes all the time that I realised how much I love Garri, a very cheap food in comparison. I had discussions with a friend in the UK who I sent Garri to and he confirmed this love when he said and I quote. 'Even if you send me to Buckingham Palace to stay with the queen, I will still eat Garri'. Why are we so attached to Garri a food not for the rich but for the masses?

We are attached because it was a top up food as people in boarding houses who often had little to eat. We are attached to it as West Africans because it is made from a staple tuber, cassava. I can say without equivocation that if Meghan was raised in Ghana she would have introduce Prince Harry to the eating of Garri. When it comes to food Garri is a stronghold on the taste buds of West Africans.

PRAYER NUGGETS

Strongholds of the Mind

1) Strongholds are places dominated by a particular group or characteristics because it is a fortification of safety for them to thrive.

2) What takes your attention is what is on your mind and as long as it occupies your mind you will soon act on it.

3) Our character is a set of predictable reactions we show in actions and emotions when we encounter certain situations in life.

4) Habits are repeated behaviours or tendencies which have been practised for so long that they are now on autopilot: they happen without our conscious thought.

CHAPTER 2

ADDICTION

Introduction

Addiction is a brain disorder characterized by compulsive engagement in rewarding stimuli despite adverse consequences. Addictions are things we take or behaviours we get involved with because of the rewards it brings to our brain. Addictions are simply a chase for the thrill till the brain's rewards system gets overloaded so it begin to think it needs it all the time. Every addiction starts as an activity to give us a thrill or satisfy curiosity but end up continuing obsessively despite the damage it might be causing us emotionally or physically.

Activities which produces the feel good effect, if sufficiently done or the right doses are taken, can get anyone addicted. An addiction is managing through consistent practice or in sufficient quantities to rewire the brain to consider such activities to be needed for survival. The brain then sets the engagement in that action or the taking of such substances as a must and therefore fight it when interventions are made to stop them. The body's' rejections of the actions to redeem it from addictions are what is normally called a state of withdrawal.

There are Six (6) main types of addictions namely: Extreme ideology Addictions; Relationship Addictions; Behavioural Addictions; Substance Addictions; Sexual Addiction and Demon Induced Addictions.

1) Substance Addiction

Dependence on drugs like cocaine, LDS, nicotine, opioid, Amphetamine, food and alcohol shall be referred to as substance addiction. These drugs initially bring relief from pressure and may even embolden users to be able to do things that they would ordinarily not be able to do.

There many artistes in the entertainment industry who turned to drugs to be able to muster the stamina and composures to be able to stand in front of large crowds for hours. Others tried substances which they though were for pure pleasure and ended up getting hooked to them. Others use substances as coping mechanism during times of sadness or stress. There many people who are addicted to food but are not aware: though it is making them sick. There are others who eat all kinds of strange things without a nutritional benefit because it helped then deal with certain emotions at certain difficult time in the lives. Most young people drink themselves to death whilst others who are born again and tongues speaking usually eat themselves to death. Some women develop strange eating habits during pregnancies or when their husbands' attention is on other women.

2) Relationship Addictions

There are many people in relationships which are not helping them but they do not want to get out of it. They are addicted to the idea of being with that particular person, because of what he or she makes them feel or the image the person accords them. There are people who are in physically abusive relationships who say it is the best relationship for them.

There are even women I know who claim that sex after the man has begged for forgiveness after beating her is the best kind of sex. There are men who seem to be addicted to married woman or pregnant women. There are others whose addictions are relationships with members of the same sex, with animals or even both. Others are addicted to relationships with children or with people old enough to be their parent or grandparent. Many of these people will tell you of the physical trauma they have to endure for these relationship choices yet they are unwilling or unable to stop. People are addicted to relationships where they are always the gold diggers or relationships where they are always the providers whether male or female. There are others who are addicted to certain actresses or actors, imagining them as wives or husbands respectively. This is also called fantasy relationships: they then seek that kind of relationship from their partners forgetting the actors were just playing a role in that production.

Thirteen (13) Reconstructive surgeries

I read about a girl who had gone through over thirteen cosmetic surgeries just to look like the actress Angelina Jolie. Her relationship with her as an actress has gone to appoint where she believes she is her and so must look like her.

There are also others who are addicted to watching others have sex. They do this because they relate to such people as avatars they control in their minds to live their fantasies. This addiction is expressed mostly in teenage boys or single young men through pornography. In their imaginations they are the ones involved in the sexual act they are watching. There are many men who are so hooked to these porn actors that they do not find their wives sexually attractive anymore. When the addiction gets out of hand such people then force their spouses to sleep with others so they can watch. What depravity! The extent to which man can fall when he loses control of himself to lust or the devil is baffling. Others are so addicted to seeing porn actors changing partners that they engage in wife swapping with others who are equally depraved to satisfy their addiction.

3) Behavioural Addictions

One of the commonest types of behavioural addiction is gambling. Gambling is a very common addiction around the world. The Chinese are known to be particularly prone to this addiction gambling billions in Macau each year. The gambling capital of the United States is Les Vegas where casino owners make billions from widows to multibillionaires who are addicted to gambling.

Gambling is so effective for rubbing people of billions that countries in the developed world and even others in the developing world use it as a means to raise revenue for the state. Gambling at casinos is not the only kind of gambling addiction, any form of decision making which is based on chance only is gambling. Why is gambling destructive? It is bad because once addicted you will sell your babies drugs for a fix of gambling. People have gambled their entire inheritance away being solely motivated by the fact that, there is a chance they may win the next one. Most places where poverty is endemic, it is so because people there are plagued with gambling their opportunities away because they are mostly waiting for a great chance to move them out of poverty instead of putting pragmatic steps in place to solve problems.

Many gamble with their lives away still believing there is the chance that they will make it elsewhere in the world. They see people drowning and dying of thirst in the desert yet they believe on chance alone that they will survive and on chance again that when they survive they will have prosperous lives in the West. Others with hope not chance are using scholarships and their talents to make the same journey albeit through airports and embassies.

I have watched documentaries on people who attempted this journey through the desert, made it to Europe but were kept in detention and subsequently deported back to their countries after wasting years, still nursing the idea of going back through the desert again. This cannot be determination but the repeat act of an addict. This is clearly a matter that is beyond desperation because as they travel they usually have thousands of dollars with them yet they will convince themselves they are desperately poor. Eh! The power of addictions to blind you against the obvious.

Apart from gambling we also have addictions for gaming, shopping, extreme attention seeking, Risky or dangerous sports etc.

4) **Sexual addictions**.

Sexual addictions are some' of the most pervasive of all addictions in this generation. People due to abuse, parental negligence, wrong company or wrong friends have developed all kinds of sexual perversions. There are people who are addicted to sleeping with animals or with people of the same sex. There are people addicted to sleeping with men and women. People who are addicted to a lot of sexual rounds in a day not necessarily because they enjoy it so much but because they think they need it to feel satisfied.

There are people addicted to sleeping with themselves using their own hands or objects. There are people who are addicted to the kind of sex which inflicts pain. Strangely there are even others who want to be physically abused during sex. There is a hotel in Eastern Europe which provides animal prostitutes for people to come and sleep with. People have died of diseases, lost marriages, been killed by jealous lovers, and even lost their means of livelihood because of sexual addictions.

I once watched a documentary where a young man was so addicted to masturbation that he could not even keep a job. He kept going to the bathroom every thirty minutes or even less to engage in this practise whenever he saw a nice young woman. He ejaculated so often that he always felt weak and was unable to work for long hours.

5) **Extreme or Fanatical ideological Addictions**

This is a strange one: people who tend to drift always to the extreme. People who need 'a we against them message'. These people thrive on 'a we against them' situation and believe in having enemies for them to progress their faith or beliefs. People who need some extreme regime to feel they are serving God. People who are so extreme that they are willing to kill others who are not righteous by their standards. People who are ready to die or kill for their understanding of God. It is an addiction which plagues entire religions and regions in the world. People who deny themselves of everything just because according to them God requires their sacrifice to complete the finished work of Christ on the cross.

Such people always see the world as sinful and depraved. To the extreme ideological addict, any actions they take on behalf of their faith is justified, no matter how crude or gruesome. We see ideological addicts burning themselves and their congregation because the world is unworthy of them, breaking away from a perfectly fine church because the leader is losing focus or forming cults to practise an extreme form of their belief. These addict believe crawling on your needs in prayer till your needs bleed is a better way to pray than sincerely taking your needs before your father in heaven. Are you aware there are Christians who fasted for so long that it led to their deaths? God is not a wicked master who loves to see us suffer before he helps as, everything he encourages as to do is for our own spiritual and physical development.

6) Demons induced Addictions

Things of the spirit are more powerful than things of the flesh. The Bible attests to it when it says that things of the spirit are eternal but things of the flesh are temporal. There are demons in charge of the various addictions. Like anything which steals, destroys and kills the devil has agents in charge of addictions. The unbelievers can therefore be afflicted by demons of addiction to engage in one perversion or the other. I know testimonies of people who were drunkards or addicted to nicotine who after deliverance could not even stand the scent of alcohol or nicotine.

If you grew up in Africa then I am sure you have head people confessing as former witches that they placed the wrong sexual desires upon their victims so they will be sexual perverts. People who went for help from the occult or fetishes and soon began to have strange sexual desires they had never experienced before till then.

Let us go to the next section where we will discuss how each addiction creates dependence within the addict and how that dependence then alters the life he or she lives. There are five ways dependency is created in the addict. They have been explained in the chapters in section two. The first chapter under this section considers how Substance addictions creates substance dependence and the forms they take.

PRAYER NUGGETS

Addictions

1) Addiction is a brain disorder characterized by compulsive engagement in rewarding stimuli despite adverse consequences.

2) There are Six (6) main types of addictions: Extreme ideology addiction; Relationship Addictions; Behavioural Addictions; Substance Addictions; Sexual Addiction and Demon Induced Addictions.

3) The most widely known addictions are sexual additions and substance addictions.

4) There are other addictions that are not common, especially in developing countries like Relationship Addiction and Extreme Ideology addiction

SECTION II: ADDICTION INDUCED DEPENDANCE

CHAPTER 3

SUBSTANCE DEPENDANCE

Dependence is reliance on something or someone because of the crucial role it or they plays in your life. It can also be a thing which plays an indispensable role in your life. The nature of dependable things or people is that, they are always around when you need them and hardly fail to give you the support you need.

The whole point of dependence is reliability or continual availability. In this context we will take the following definitions of dependence: the state of being conditional or contingent on something, as through a natural or logical sequence; the dependence of an effect upon a cause; the state of being psychologically or physiologically dependent on a drug after a prolonged period of use (Dictionary.com, 2018).

Dependence on food

Proverbs 23:21 King James Version (KJV)

21 For the drunkard and the glutton shall come to poverty: and drowsiness shall clothe a man with rags.

There are many who eat as a means to assuage painful emotions they are failing to deal with. People who eat because they are lonely or angry. This dependence on food as a solution to emotional or relationship problems becomes a problem in itself because more food is eaten than the body can process. Repeatedly eating as a way to take the pain of offense or heartbreak will not solve the problem but rewire the brain to love instructing you to eat when you are not hungry.

The brain will be tricked to think you need to overeat all the time to be happy. Eating too much will affect your weight and health leading to sadness or hurtful comments from friends and loved ones which will induced more eating. The cycle of addictions is then complete and takes a life of its own outside the conscious decisions of the addict to eat or not to eat. So longs as the conditions are right the person will have little resistance eating something to feel good about himself or herself. Mostly the activity will be so far from the person mind that most people will deny engaging in it.

An addict only owns up to his or her addictions when the havoc it is causing becomes obvious.

Dependence on alcohol

As proverbs 23:21 clearly teaches alcohol and gluttony wastes our resources. Addictions lead the addict into repeated expenditures which do not improve his or her welfare in any way. Expenditures which over time increase in frequency and quantum. Most people around the world use alcohol to escape the realities of live: the loneliness, the sadness, and the fear of taking certain importance decisions. Interestingly people in the very developed part of south East Asia are known to be addicts to alcohol. Many people pick this addiction when they are under stress or are grieving.

The repeated use of alcohol to numb the pain they feel in their hearts leads to behavioural or attitudinal changes which provokes negative commentaries from friends, colleagues and relatives leading to more sadness   and loneliness. This forms a reinforcing cycle: where the sadness leads to more drinking and the drinking due to adverse behavioural changes leads to more sadness.

Dependence on smoking, injectable or tablets

People usually get involved in using nicotine, injectable or tablets because of peer pressure. And they usually yield to this pressures because they want to belong or fit into the group. Others start using these substance because they want to demonstrate that they are trendy or tough. Many people also use these to calm their nerves when they are anxious or about to appear before a crowd. These are generally referred to as recreational drugs and are used as experience enhancers. Some produce the bold, good, strong, cool feeling amongst especially the school going teens or youth.

They usually use these drugs whenever they want to invoke these feelings of invincibility as teens or young adults. In the developed world people experiment with this at the universities and colleges the most. Cigarettes are considered as the gateway drugs which lead to others like marijuana, sniffing of cocaine, taking of tablets and injectable. These drugs have the ability to alter your reality, tricking the brain to believe things which are not real. The bliss associated with taking those tablets, sniffing that powder or smoking that weed provides the push for it to be used again and again.

The addiction cycle involves the bliss it provides to the user. Then with time the user will need to use more at frequent times to experience the same bliss as the first time. In that way more is used till the body becomes depended on it for survival.

These drugs mind altering power can destroy your ability to reason and may lead to cancers or madness. Discontinuing the use of these drugs is very difficult because of the painful withdrawal symptoms it imposes on the addict.

Dependence on Things or Drugs Which Make Us Feel Good

Addiction does not always start with abuse of illicit drugs like heroin. In fact, prescription narcotic analgesics -- pain medications that have been legally prescribed to a patient from a healthcare provider -- sits at the heart of the U.S. epidemic of fatal overdoses (Anderson, 2018).

There is an epidemic of prescription drugs addiction in the United States and other western countries. Many people in these developed countries are suffering from pains of all kinds: from migraines, surgeries, old age and from broken heart or abusive relationships. The drugs which use to help these people to deal with their pains have become a need for their systems and is now needed for them to function normally as individuals.

Many of these people have found ways of obtaining opioids or narcotics painkillers in greater quantities than they need. Many repeat this practice more often than is allowed.

Thus in less than six months they get high on these otherwise harmless medicines. There are others who developed the habits of chewing clay or some other materials when they were pregnant to control nausea but are now dependent of it even after giving birth. Many people are hooked to pills or bitters for improve sexual performance but are failing to realise it is affecting the organs in their bodies.

There are people who cannot function unless they have strong perfume on. They need to wear a strong perfume or smell a particular way to be confident outside of the house. The wig industry in Africa is about six billion dollars in turn over annually, because there are many women in Africa who are addicted to wearing a wigs to feel beautiful or properly dressed. Women who never show their natural hair because years or watching women in wigs or European woman has made them an addict to wigs.

There are women who are addicted to makeup and will never step out of the house without heavy makeup. Such people use permanent makeups so they will not be caught often without it. All these being people who have fallen victim to the lies of

Hollywood where a woman comes out of the pool with makeup and even wakes up from the bed with makeup.

Because the image they come out with is not natural so they need to go everywhere with it so as to keep that image before funs or the husband they marry later in their career.

PRAYER NUGGETS

Dependence on Substance

1) Addictions is dependence on substance, relationship or an emotions which is destroying your life.

2) Substances that people are addicted to include: food, prescription drugs and alcohol.

3) Other substances people abuse are: LSD, Cocaine, Heroin, Crystal Meth, Marijuana etc.

4) People become addicted to substance which once relieved their pain, made them feel good or even quench their test.

CHAPTER 4

DEPENDANCE ON A RELATIONSHIP

Depends on a relationship to feel whole or complete

There are people who are suffering all kinds of abuse from their spouses or partners yet they believe they are in the best of relationships. These people have become so dependent on the desires or gifts the partner is lavishing that they are more than happy to endure the verbal and physical abuse from their partner or spouse. Like many cases of dependence, this addict will initially be isolated from all her supports systems and made only to need this partner or spouse.

As the years passes she grows to source all her emotional and even material needs from him and him only. She is now addicted to him and what he gives her. No amount of persuasion from friends at this stage will help her back out of the relationship. She will use his past kindness, her poor background, the fact that her abusive partner will change and so on as excuses to stay in the relationship till one day her body is found somewhere in the house.

Dependent on a relationship to feel appreciated or respected

David was a victim of relationship addiction: Michal the daughter of Saul had a crush on David, the shepherd boy who had overnight become the saviour of Israel. Saul sees an opportunity to keep David on leash through his daughter and offers her to him with tax free benefits for himself and his family. All these Saul did to get David into an abusive relationship: a relationship where David will always feel indebted to his spouse and in laws.

1 Samuel 18:20-21 King James Version (KJV)

20 And Michal Saul's daughter loved David: and they told Saul, and the thing pleased him. 21 And Saul said, I will give him her, that she may be a snare to him, and that the hand of the Philistines may be against him. Wherefore Saul said to David, Thou shalt this day be my son in law in the one of the twain.

David saw it as promotion but Saul saw it as a trap which will eventually cut short his life. Michal was eventually given to another man whilst David was running for his life.

The marriage that was supposed to make David and his family in-laws to the first king of Israel ended up endangering their lives. David thought he was getting a trophy wife but ended up with a secret weapon of Saul which almost destroyed his life. Like any addiction David still longed for Michal even after tasting success without her for years and sent for her to be taken from her new husband as soon as he could.

2 Samuel 3:14-16 King James Version (KJV)

14 And David sent messengers to Ishbosheth Saul's son, saying, Deliver me my wife Michal, which I espoused to me for an hundred foreskins of the Philistines. And Ishbosheth sent, and took her from her husband, even from Phaltiel the son of Laish. 16 And her husband went with her along weeping behind her to Bahurim. Then said Abner unto him, Go, return. And he returned.

Whilst many people were running to King David during the time he was running for his dear life, Michal his wife refused to run to him. Michal the Daughter of Saul who could have made that decision with less consequences than all those who did. She happily married another man whilst David was pursued like a common criminal. She turned her new husband into another addict, getting him so drank on needing her that he cried after her as they were taking her to David.

Dependent on a particular person to feel safe or secure

There are those who have so longed to be with a particular person that they are willing to bear anything for that relationship to remain. People who are addicted to particular people because of certain body features or certain skills they possess. Someone might say that this is the 'love is blind stage' no it is not, because people in such relationships will complain about all the pain they are going through and speak frankly about the bad habits of such people.

But will still not leave them, not even after serious injuries from their assaults or after catching that spouse cheating on them on several occasions. The false sense of security or safety they feel is so strong that they convince themselves that it is worth the pain and suffering they are going through.

Testifying against Her mother

I know of a young woman who got addicted to a man like that: a man she probably met when she was far too young. He made such an impression on her that he could beat her mercilessly for any reason which came to his mind but she still kept to him against her entire family's advice. He could even beat her because she was the one supporting him instead of him supporting her and their children.

He will beat her sometimes till she runs to her mother's house and he will follow her even there to continue the beating right in front of her mother. A woman he had not even married officially. And yet when the mother sent him to court for domestic assault this girl became a defendant against her own mother till the case was struck out.

Depends On Strange Relationships to Punish Parents

Another relationship dependency which is often exhibited by especially ladies is the penchant for them to marry or date someone the parents do not like so as to spite them. Did I hear you say this is childish! Yes more than that, children who have gotten so used to upsetting their parents over the years for reason of neglect or abandonment etc. People who get into relationships which will always put them in the spotlight before their parents.

Spoilt children who use their exotic choice of partners or unconventional relationships to embarrass their parents who are often traditional in outlook and powerful or rich. People addicted to showing they are the black sheep of the family in the people they choose to date or even marry. These sort of addicts are found especially in the homes of successful pastors.

Pastors who committed more of their time to ministry instead of raising their children. Esau's prospects in life were reduce drastically because he felt the need to live up to the reputation of being a wild man and married without his parents' consent, the daughters of Canaan to the chagrin of his parents. No wonder his mother plotted against him with his brother to steal his blessings

Genesis 27:46 King James Version (KJV)

46 And Rebekah said to Isaac, I am weary of my life because of the daughters of Heth: if Jacob take a wife of the daughters of Heth, such as these which are of the daughters of the land, what good shall my life do me?

Sampson's addiction to strange women ended his ministry and eventually his life. Though Sampson was the strongest man who ever lived he could not fight the dangers that dating strange women all the time brought to him. He was an addict to the women of the Philistines and would not heed his parents call for him to date women from Israel till it killed him

Judges 16:1, 2,4,19 King James Version (KJV)

1Then went Samson to Gaza, and saw there an harlot, and went in unto her. And it was told the Gazites, saying, Samson is come hither. 2 And they compassed him in, and laid wait for him all

night in the gate of the city, and were quiet all the night, saying, In the morning, when it is day, we shall kill him. 4 And it came to pass afterward, that he loved a woman in the valley of Sorek, whose name was Delilah.19 And she made him sleep upon her knees; and she called for a man, and she caused him to shave off the seven locks of his head; and she began to afflict him, and his strength went from him.

Depends On a Relationship to Avert Loneliness or Fear of Losing a Soul Mate

There are many people especially women who are addicted to the African Movies type of husband or partner who looks immaculate and is ready to overlook every misdeed of theirs whilst literally lifting them of their feet with gifts and lots of pampering. Men who will always admire them no matter what time of day it is and be around most of the time to spend 'quality time' with them. However these men will also have to be financially sound to 'spoil them' every now and then with trips to lovely places.

The addiction or craze for a soul mate and the romantic demands which is expected of them has created three different breed of men: men who are romantic and financially sound but not faithful; men who are romantic and faithful, mostly Christian but not financially sound at the beginning; and last but not least men who are passionate lovers but neither faithful nor financially sound. These addicts to 'movie love' therefore jump from one relationship to the next with the expectation of securing the perfect match.

Others keep going back to that first man or woman in spite of all the wrongs in that relationship because somehow they believe he or she could be their soul mate. The only reason someone keeps going back to something or someone which is physically or mentally destructive is because he or she is addicted to it, him or her.

The condition where people feel lonely unless they are with a particular person in spite of all the love ones and relatives who surround them is an addiction. Situations where people think they have to lie or 'go under the knife' to be able to keep or attract that soul mate is clearly a sign of an addiction.

Husband in a dustbin

I heard something from a friend of mine which clearly illustrates this point of addiction to 'movie star love' or the 'African movies type romance'. He told me he has a female friend who has been properly married to a responsible husband.

But this lady once remarked to him that whenever she watches the kind of love men show to their wives in the movies and the appearance of such men, she wished she could pick her husband, the man who is the head of her household and put him in a dustbin and close it.

The movie husband in the movies she has been watching are so good that in comparison her husband's efforts and appearance look like rubbish to be put in a dustbin. She has forgotten to add that she in no way appears and act like the actresses in those movies but thinks she deserves those actors, an obvious omission she is failing to see like any other addict would.

PRAYER NUGGETS

Dependence on a relationship

1) People are said to be addicted to a relationship when that relationship is destroying their life yet they do not want to end it.

2) The relationship no more persist as a result of love when the abused partner admits the abuse and yet offer reasons other than wellbeing to continue the relationship.

3) People are dependent on a relationship because it gives them respect or make them feel secure.

4) Others are addicted to a relationship because they believe they are their 'soul mate' or because they do not want to be lonely.

CHAPTER 5

DEPENDANCE ON AN EMOTION OR FEELING

Introduction

King Solomon was addicted to feeling great and had a desire for more pleasure all the time. He went out of his way to pursue it till it became an addiction which almost ruined his kingdom. His emotions drove him to have relationships with about a thousand women from all the nations of the ancient world. Those same emotions drove the wisest man who ever lived to act foolishly: His addictions drove him to the worshipping foreign gods because he wanted to please his many lovers.

1 Kings 11:1-6 King James Version (KJV)

11 But king Solomon loved many strange women, together with the daughter of Pharaoh, women of the Moabites, Ammonites, Edomites, Zidonians, and Hittites: 2 Of the nations concerning which the Lord said unto the children of Israel, Ye shall not go in to them, neither shall they come in unto you: for surely they will turn away your heart after their gods: Solomon clave unto these in love. 3 And he had seven hundred wives, princesses, and three hundred concubines: and his wives turned away his heart. 4 For it came to pass, when Solomon was old, that his wives turned away his heart after other gods: and his heart was not perfect with the Lord his God, as was the heart of David his father. 5 For Solomon went after Ashtoreth the goddess of the Zidonians, and after Milcom the abomination of the Ammonites. 6 And Solomon did evil in the sight of the Lord, and went not fully after the Lord, as did David his father.

Dependent on feelings of optimism after abuse

There are people who are addicted to the emotion of optimism. They get a rush when there is a glimmer of hope even after years of frustration. They are addicted to the feeling of being right that it was worth hoping for the best. Such people will remain in hopeless situations or relationships just because they cannot stop being optimistic that things will turn around.

Such people will keep giving birth with a man who has refused to work or a woman who is a chronic adulteress. Anytime this spouse will shed tears after being caught in the act once again the addict will see it a sign of a recovery and get an emotional rush to stay, though it will not amount to much.

If you are a pastor or friend to such a person all your pieces of advice will fall on death ears till the person's life is destroyed or worse killed by this incorrigible partner.

Dependent on the Feeling of Bliss after Violent Abuse

There are others who are addicted to the feeling of bliss and will endure anything to have it from time to time. The bliss the feel after passionate love making from a 'repented' spouse or lover who just violently assaulted them.

And before you think such a person will be an illiterate nobody, let me shock you, there are highly educated professional men and women in this situation too. Famous people who are so addicted to the emotions of bliss that they even enjoy being beaten before intimacy because it heightens their emotion if bliss. Women who swear that sex after being beaten or what they usually call make up sex is the best kind of sex.

Dependent on the Feeling of Sadness

There are people who because of their abusive childhood do not feel alive unless they are sad .These emotional addicts will look for every opportunity to be sad, no matter how remote.

There are women who are sad because they believe they do not deserve the love being shown them by their partners. Others are sad for reasons the average woman will jump for joy: that their husband feel obligated to stay around far too often. Such people's favourite lie is that: they are having tears of joy.

These sad souls are at their best during funerals, they will usually cry even more than the closest relatives of the deceased because they just love the attention being sad brings to them. Many of these people grew up in families where only sadness and tears could get things done and have obviously become addicted to it over the years.

Dependent on the Emotion of Being Right All the Time

These I am always right addicts are a handful in any relationship: they must be right in every argument and will used all kinds of emotions to achieve it, if necessary. They get frustrated when their point of view is not taken and will result to all kinds of emotional manoeuvring, show of signs of frustration and anger to ensure they carry the day. Spouses of such people will either have to say yes to everything they say or face endless quarrels because they must be right all the time.

Such addicts enjoy such great emotions when they win an argument, a fix they need to have from time to time. Such people grew up having everything to themselves and have been groomed to believe they are more intelligent than the average person. These addicts enjoy telling everyone how right they always are against how wrong everyone's opinion or action is, relative to theirs.

Please pray that you do not encounter such a person as your boss. These people poison everyone's opinion of them till they are left practically alone yet they still believe their attitude or emotional disposition is the best. I am sure you are not surprised to hear that. Because you dear reader, has encountered one of these people before.

Dependent on Others Feeling Sad To Be Happy

Unhappy people are often relieved to see they are not the only ones in that situation. But others take this tendency even further: if you could see into the hearts of people who are your colleagues, team mates and even relatives you will be shocked to know the extent to which people want you to fail so they can be happy. I dare say that for every progress a man or woman makes there are more people who are sad than those who are happy.

I am not talking 'rival happiness' which result from a team beating the rival but deep seated need in people to see you sad so they can feel happy.

Psychologist describe such people as sociopathic, sadistic, or psychopathic. People with this addiction can easily sink into violence or terrorism. Marrying people with this addiction is mostly hell on earth: because he or she will enjoy seeing you suffer for one reason or the other most of the time.

PRAYER NUGGETS

Dependence on an Emotion or Feeling

1) People become dependent on an emotion or feeling when they know it is causing them harm yet they cannot stop themselves from going back to it.

2) People are addicted to the emotions of bliss during reconciliation romance after physical abuse by their partners because they believe in their heart that they won him or her back.

3) People get a 'high' or a fix when they see others are sad or in trouble.

4) People are addicted to the feeling of sadness so much that they love being the victim or the disadvantaged most of the time.

CHAPTER 6

EXTREME OR FANATICAL IDEOLOGICAL ADDICTION

Introduction

Fanaticism is a wildly excessive or irrational devotion, dedication, or enthusiasm (Collin English Dictionary, 2014). An ideology on the other hand is a set of doctrines or beliefs that are shared by the members of a social group or that form the basis of a political, economic, or any other system (American Heritage® Dictionary, 2016).[8]

Fanatism in the context of an ideology is a wildly excessive or irrational set of doctrines or beliefs of a person or a group. It simply expresses the fact that people have excessive beliefs or convictions based on an irrational enthusiasm.

In this chapters we go into why fanatics are all addicts to their own version of right and wrong. Today's world call Christians who are spending and are ready to be spent for their God and the charge He has given them as fanatics.

Fanatism as an addiction or ideology is best expressed when a group of people hold onto a set of believes because it justifies their right to trample upon others for their individual or collective glory. Fanatic addict says, I only understand it this way because understanding it any other way will change my exalted position in society. Fanatic addicts are found in all faiths or beliefs. This book attempts to expose them and the dangerous religions, sects and cults they have created since the time of Nimrod the mighty warrior.

Fanatics are addicted to their own version of right

Imagine someone saying that because someone is a homosexual he has the right to rape him. What he is actually saying is that I hate this guy for sleeping with a man so much that I going to sleep with him too to teach him a lesson. Only an addict will think this line of thinking is justified. How can you perpetuate the very act you are condemning as punishment.

In the same way no Christian has the right to murder a homosexual because only dead gods need men to exact their punishment for them. See a religion which is built on fanatism and you will soon realise the adherents are quick to kill in the name of their god. Fanatism completely rejects opposition to their views.

Fanatics are addicted to their own version of right and will fight to the death to support it. God is a wise God he never instructs us to do things which are unreasonable. Faith is based on something, thus the word of God. That is why faith is not fanatism. Being reasonable does not mean being scientific but means it has been objectively analysed and the idea found to be right. In such cases your spirit will bear witness that it is true.

Religious Fanatics Have Been Brainwashed To Preserve Their Version of Right

Many ideological addicts were brain washed very early in life and are often taught using religious codes whilst being isolated from other members of the society with diverging views. Through root learning or constant repetitions of the tenets of the faith such ideas are imbibed. After much repetition of what is right and what is wrong according to that religion, sect or cult, the mind gets set on them and will not change no matter the contrary evidence provided.

Dear reader, I am not talking about devotion, for devotion considers both the letter and the spirit of the scriptures being followed.

A set of believes which says our God spoke once here in this book or on that tablet and has since left us to figure things out for ourselves is not a living religion but a dead one. A living God gives his blueprint in scriptures but still provides day to day guidance in its interpretation as the years go by to his servants. Because the use of words and their meaning change over time and needs a living God to keep speaking to bring clarity on what was said before.

Ideological addicts believe in grey and blank

Fanatics are also in the scientific community, people who dismiss the existence of God because it makes humans look weak and accountable to something beyond themselves. Such people who call themselves agnostic and atheist believe in anything from a renowned scientist who followed the scientific method but are quick to dismiss others for believing in what their church leaders say.

Such people create the impression that a belief in God is an upfront to science as though the early scientist were not God fearing. There are many ideological addicts who are ready to believe in parallel universe and aliens but not in God and his angels. In this they show they are believers in science and not the God of the Bible.

But like most addicts they will deny they are believers and claim they are scientist instead as though there is a difference between the two. Example, before scientist set out on any scientific quest they start with a belief which when it is put in the scientific context becomes a theory. It is just a belief expressed in the understanding of scientist that is why it needs to be tested for it to be finally accepted.

The all is grey ideology addict has no convictions, the agnostic is not sure what to belief, and there in nothing out there atheist is so afraid to believe that he is ready to equate reality to only the things he can see, if he cannot see then it does not exit. What arrogance!

A mere man who does not even know how he sleeps or wakes every day wants to determine reality. Again atheist say: if I cannot proof it scientifically then it does not exist. But the gap between 'I cannot prove God' and the fact that He God exist is pure belief and not a product of the scientific method.

Ideological Addicts Are Bullies Using Emotions to Cover the Lack of Facts or Truth to Back Their Beliefs

These are the people who result to violence and threats when they run out of truth to defend their religion. People who do not follow other people's way of life yet call for others who do not follow their religion to be killed because they have offended them in something they said. How can a merciful God inspire so much hatred in his followers for people who need saving or redeeming. The Bible prescribes the best way to avoid contention with unbelievers: do not retaliate.

But the carnally minded says it is not reasonable, the reasonable approach is rather to attack them first because they have offended us. Only an addict can think such an excessive approach is reasonable. Such people are made to feel they are right so long as they go through the motions and performs the various rites. And as far as their actions go to defend their faith against unbelievers they are justified.

If righteousness was doing what you like to those who do not like you then the unbelievers are more righteous because they outnumber the believers but do not mobilise to attack us. As young people watch what you think and how you think before you get hook to an idea which will ruin your lives in the future. Study indeed to show yourself approved as a young man or woman who needs not to be ashamed.

Those who might not be religion inclined might express their insistence or the fact that they are right all the time through video games, where they refuse to stop playing till they win.

A couple in South Korea kept feeding their virtual baby in a game for three days non-stop and left their real baby to starve to death in their flat. They could not stop to attending to the virtual baby and lose the game so they sacrificed their real baby to continue the game. Video game addiction also falls under this kind of addiction where people want to win at all cost.

2 Timothy 2:15 King James Version (KJV)

15 Study to shew thyself approved unto God, a workman that needeth not to be ashamed, rightly dividing the word of truth.

PRAYER NUGGETS

Extreme or Fanatical ideological addictions

1) People are ideological addicts if they believe only the most extreme form of a religion is right: especially if it humiliates followers or call for the killing of unbelievers.
2) Ideological addicts believe in grey and blank instead of white and black.
3) Ideological addicts have their own version of right and are prepared to die or kill for it.
4) Ideological addicts or fanatics use fear and intimidation to cover for their lack of facts to communicate their beliefs adequately.

CHAPTER 7

FIXATED ON A DESIRE

Background

The Roman church in biblical times was like the churches in the developed world today. Churches in the midst of people who believe in their achievements as men, to be enough for them. People proud of the achievements of their ancestors and proud of their citizenship of Rome or in this instance a first world country. Who are steeped in materialism and superstition: believe in Santa clause and aliens but have rejected the creator of the universe. People consumed by their own version of what the right or wrong worldview is.

People only interested in the pleasures of this world and uninterested in where they will spend eternity. To counter this attitude toward God, Paul wrote to make it clear to the people of Rome that their environment and desires have given them over to sinful and unnatural pleasures which will eventually destroy them.

Romans 1:26-31 King James Version (KJV)

26 For this cause God gave them up unto vile affections: for even their women did change the natural use into that which is against nature: 27 And likewise also the men, leaving the natural use of the woman, burned in their lust one toward another; men with men working that which is unseemly, and receiving in themselves that recompense of their error which was meet. 28 And even as they did not like to retain God in their knowledge, God gave them over to a reprobate mind, to do those things which are not convenient; 29 Being filled with all unrighteousness, fornication, wickedness, covetousness, maliciousness; full of envy, murder, debate, deceit, malignity; whisperers, 30 Backbiters, haters of God, despiteful, proud, boasters, inventors of evil things, disobedient to parents, 31 Without understanding, covenant breakers, without natural affection.

King Solomon was fixated on the desire to experience anything desirable in this world. These addictions brought untold hardship to the people he governed and led him to many strange practices and idols of his wives in his old age.

Ecclesiastes 2 King James Version (KJV)

10 And whatsoever mine eyes desired I kept not from them, I withheld not my heart from any joy; for my heart rejoiced in all my labour: and this was my portion of all my labour.11 Then I looked on all the works that my hands had wrought, and on the labour that I had laboured to do: and, behold, all was vanity and vexation of spirit, and there was no profit under the sun.

Man is mostly driven by his convictions and his dominant desires. Every desire man focuses on grows. Jesus validates this truth when he illustrated the power of a fixated desire by saying it is the same as doing the act in your heart. He said, if you fix your desires on sleeping with a woman you meet on the street you will end up having a release in your body as though you actually slept with her. You would not have physically touched her but in your heart you would have undressed her and committed adultery or fornication with her.

Matthew 5:28 King James Version (KJV)

28 But I say unto you, That whosoever looketh on a woman to lust after her hath committed adultery with her already in his heart.

The phrase 'look on a woman to lust' is an illustration of a fixated desire to have sex with a woman, albeit in your heart.

It does not mean a man noticing a woman is beautiful or attractive; but a man focusing sexual desire on a woman to a points of sexual satisfaction in his heart. If you ask the average teenager who is not born again, they will share with you times when they lusted so much for a pretty woman in real life, movie or picture that they reached orgasm and ejaculated as if they were physically with her. For the man or woman who undergoes this process, Jesus says you have committed adultery with her in your heart. This has the same spiritual implication as though you actually did sleep with her.

Unnatural Desire or lust for sex

Lust is a craving or an overwhelming desire for sex. The desire for sex is natural but the desire for sex all the time is not. .The desire for sex with any beautiful woman or handsome man is not natural either. The desire for someone of the same sex is also not natural. Even worse is the sexual desire of animals.

All wrong forms of sexual cravings are addictions either caught or taught. Taught in the sense that you were forced to endure it in times past and your brain has rewired itself to think that you need it or you caught it through demonic afflictions.

People addicted to the cravings for unnatural sex do so because of the blissful experience they feel when they engage in that activity though many become depressed soon afterwards. A sign that their soul is unhappy with their lifestyle: suicide and sexual transmitted disease rates are higher amongst gays and lesbians than heterosexuals.

Similarly, people involved in prostitution are also prone to depression and have higher rate of contracting sexually transmitted diseases. Addiction to sexual desires has caused the fall of many great men and has even prematurely ended the lives of others from the scandal which ensued. It has also destroyed many families and have given many strange women power over men of God.

Extreme Desire for Attention

There are people who because of parental neglect or other childhood abuses have a strong craving for attention. Such people will alter any uniform you give them such that it will draw attention wherever they pass. Like children they will paint their hair, cars or house in very bright colours to draw attention. When you are in a relationship with such people they will expect you to talk to them all the time. They are even ready to sell their souls to the devil if it will bring fame to them.

They will get extremely incensed if every cloth, hairdo, or word they say does not draw commentary from the important people in their lives. Such people, especially the women are ready to go naked if it will bring them a lot of attention on social media. As spouses they will take decisions thinking of what will bring attention to the family without considering whether it serve their interest.

Histrionic personality disorder (HPD) is characterized by a long-standing pattern of attention seeking behaviour and extreme emotionality. Someone with histrionic personality disorder wants to be the centre of attention in any group of people, and they feel uncomfortable when they are not. While often lively, interesting, and sometimes dramatic, they have difficulty when people aren't focused exclusively on them. People with this disorder may be perceived as being shallow, and may engage in sexually seductive or provocative behaviour to draw attention to themselves (Bressert, 2017).

Desire for What Belongs To Others

Envy is the desire for what belongs to others. Woe unto you if your partner or spouse is addicted to desiring what others have or are. Such people are obsessed with what others are doing and building in their lives whilst neglecting their own lives.

They never praise anything they have unless they see it with another person. Such people are thieves, unfaithful partners and are capable of killing to take over someone's properties. The addictions of 'what is with others is better' plagues many young men and women of Africa who are risking their lives to go to Europe to seek greener pastures. This addiction is called the Greener Pastures syndrome: it afflicts the youth in many poor countries and neighbourhoods.

Deuteronomy 5:21 King James Version (KJV)

21 Neither shalt thou desire thy neighbour's wife, neither shalt thou covet thy neighbour's house, his field, or his manservant, or his maidservant, his ox, or his ass, or anything that is thy neighbour's.

The strong desires for what belongs to others to a point where you are ready to harm the person to get it, is covetousness and is the root of all witchcraft and most violence in the world. Many are addicted to this desire though the Lord forbids as from engaging in such activities. If the only time you see something is nice or good is when a friend is using it and such thoughts have persisted for a while then you need to be set free from it before it destroys your prospects in life.

An Iranian woman has gone viral after claiming she's had 50 surgeries in a bid to look like her idol Angelina Jolie. Sahar Tabar claims to be one of the "Tomb Raider" actress' biggest fans and has said she "would do anything" to emulate her. The 19-year-old from Tehran underwent 50 surgeries in the space of just a few months, according to Al Arabiya (Windle, 2017).

This woman who was already pretty but was so obsessed with looking like someone else that she ruined her looks in the end.

Addicted To the Desire for Risky Behaviours

This addiction falls under the general gambling addiction. People who think reasonable harm cannot come to them not because they are well prepared but because of chance or luck. People who take decisions believing luck will always smile at them. These people have no idea of Murphy's law which states that, if something can go wrong, then it will, no matter if you are prepared for it or not.

These people get a fix or thrill in the face of danger. They are affectionately called adrenalin junkies. They love to date dangerous men, are quick to volunteer for dangerous jobs, perilous journeys and are quick to date people they no next to nothing about. For such, the threat or danger gives them a rush that is so satisfying that they are unable to control themselves from rushing in when an opportunity presents itself.

Thrill seekers share many of the same symptoms as drug addicts; they get a rush from skydiving or rock climbing, but after a while, they seek out even more dangerous adventures to feel that same level of excitement. And studies show that these thrills flood the brain with the same chemicals released by addictive drugs (Davis, 2018).[11]

Addicted To the Desire to Shop or Get New Things

Shopping: It's yet another behaviour that, when it spins out of control, is considered to be an impulse control disorder (rather than a true addiction). Do you purchase items to avoid feeling sad — but then feel guilty afterwards? *Do you have a closet full of clothes that still have the price tags on them? You could be a shopaholic. Studies show that compulsive shopping affects more women than men, and that it can result in big problems, both financially and personally* (Davis, 2018).

There are many people who cannot keep to one relationship or interest for life. They have this uncontrollable edge to start fresh things all the time or pick new items very frequently. Such people do not go by the adage 'if it is not broke then do not fix it.' They can change the plan of their house ten times before the building is finished or change a car they are using every year whether the replacement is better or not.

Everything New

I had a colleague at work who kept buying cars, none of which was better than the first. He could buy a car just within an hour of sighting it. You are saying it is because he was very wealthy, no most of the cars he bought broke down for one reason or the other. There were times he had as many as four broken down cars at various places but had to ask friends for the use of their cars.

This permeated other parts of his life: he was never faithful to his wives or partners but kept changing women as if they were going out of fashioned. He even experimented with new religions, once he was a traditionalist then a Christian for a while and then Moslem by marriage. This addiction caused him to waste many opportunities and contributed in no small part to end his life.

PRAYER NUGGETS

Fixated on a Desire

1) There are people who are addicted to desires because such desires occupy their hearts and mind all day. These desires drive them to behaviours which bring sadness and shame yet they cannot bring themselves to stop it.

2) There are people who are addicted to the feeling of satisfaction after shopping and so are addicted to shopping for things they do not need.

3) There are others who are addicted to the thrill of escaping death in dangerous situations, adrenalin junkies who are always engaged in potential life threating sports.

4) Attentions seekers, people addicted to being the centre of attention. People who are ready to strip naked and put it on social media so long as it will bring them attention.

SECTION III: HOW PEOPLE GET ADDICTED

CHAPTER 8

PATHWAYS TO ADDICTIONS

Using Substances to Assuage Negative Emotions

One of the main ways people get addicted is through substance abuse. Examples of substances people usually abuse are drugs both hard and prescribed, alcohol, nicotine and food. The most common substances people get addicted to include: Alcohol, Amphetamine or similarly acting sympathomimetic, Benzodiazepines, Caffeine, Cannabis, Cocaine, Hallucinogens, Inhalants Nicotine, Opioids, Phencyclidine (PCP) similar acting agents, Sedatives, hypnotics or anxiolytics.

The use of substances or chemicals to generate emotions or feelings which for a moment make the individual forget his pain or frustration can lead to addiction. The gain or relief is usually short live so the process needs to be repeated fairly regularly and consistently to make a lasting impression. The brain then begins to see the relief provided as a need and begins to crave for it all the time. Whatever drug, nicotine or alcohol which provided the relief then needs to be consumed to keep the relief going until the substance becomes as needed as the initial elusive emotion or feeling sought. The addict then forgets about the initial problems because the drug or nicotine which by now needs to be taken in increasing frequency and amount to produce the safe relief it initially provided will be causing its own problems.

Using drugs to overcome fear

Fear is for flight or fight but for most people fear paralyses them and makes them incapable of doing what is expected. For most people the fear of harm, disappointment or disgrace causes them to settle for less than their soul deserves. Many people resort to the taking of drugs to boost their confidence but over time the body adjust to the amount taken leading to the effect going down.

They therefore need to take more at a frequent pace to produce the same effect of boldness anytime they are afraid. The body's need for more grows till the body begins to crave for drugs even more than the relief it brings. At this stage the fear problem would have been forgotten and the damage the drug will be causing to the body and the addict's reputation will then become the reason for concern. The original quest to deal with fear the wrong way would be bringing even more health problems. With the addicts resorting to many social vices to keep funding the habit.

Engaging In Demonic Rituals

You see celebrities using one sign or the other as they sing and you imitate them without knowing why they do them. Some of them are masonic signs to offer adoration to demons. I dare say that no one can make global impact without demonic or divine help. Many famous people are making sacrifices to the devil unknowingly with their lack of marriage, happiness, children and so on to gain fame and fortune. Children doing demonic ritual dances because they have seen them in cartoons. One of the reasons

Africa is poor though in the midst of great resources is the fact that most of our cultural practices which were rituals to please deities in the past are still being practised any time a project is being initiated. No wonder our leaders are addicted to bribery and corruption. No wonder leaders with good intention do not last but those with the most evil of intentions last for a whole generation. Some Christians are even going back to partake in ancient rituals which were dedicated to demons because of trials like lack of marriage, poverty or childlessness.

The power of casting spells or placing curses on people is common in Ghana. This has opened a lot of people to the demons of addictions as they consult fetish priests to overturn curses they cast or were sent in their direction.

Using demonic substances

Using demonic substance like Ouija boards, clothing with demonic symbols, watching demonic movies, sleeping with people anointed by demons, etc. Listening to demonic music like many hard rock where the lyrics hail the god of music and say other sacrilegious things, can open the listener to demonic attacks which can lead to all manner of addictions.

There are people who drank a demon anointed drink just one bottle and became drunkards for the rest of their lives. Just as an anointed substance empowers the Christian to achieve for the Lord in the same way a demonic material serves the cause of Satan.

At this stage dear reader give me your undivided attention, say this aloud with me as I make the following decrees: anything which the devil has put in my life or body I command it to come out in Jesus name.

I command any foreign material in my body to come out and burn in the name of Jesus Christ of Nazareth. Amen. By this prayer you have stopped evil cravings, diseases or weaknesses the devil afflicted you with in the spirit before it could manifest in the flesh.

Abuse Of Any Substance or Behaviour Consistently

Children start with practices which if not check grow to become bad habits or addictions which reduces the quality of their lives. Encouraging children to be for example fearful of the dark or to be alone starts many fear addictions in their lives. Encouraging children to use violence as a way to teach people the lessons of life stir in them violence tendencies.

The addiction of mobs to lynching bad people in countries around the world stems from this education that if people do wrong then they are deserving of death of the worst kind. Such people often believe that, it is best for the innocent to be killed so long as the guilty is not left of the hook.

This philosophy is guiding many operations of security services around the world. Now they shoot to kill first before they are shot at or killed. Many parents in a bid to keep children quiet fill their food with a lot of fatty foods, sugar or salt above the daily requirement for years. These children then grow up already addicted to these things which are responsible for most of the chronic diseases in this world today.

Mindless Imbibing of Repeated Falsehood or Propaganda

There are sons who hated the sight of their fathers beating their mothers but are now doing the same thing to their wives. Their anger or disgust as children was not powerful enough to prevent them from going the same way. Hating a practice is not enough to stop repeating it if you are exposed to it for far too long.

Because your mind will gradually be tune by the propaganda that goes with that practice day in and out from the offending parent to justify his or her actions. Girls who hated the verbal abuse of their fathers by their mothers if they do not get saved along the way, grow up to do the same thing because of the constant propaganda that they were fed with anytime they complained about the act as children growing up.

People who are addicted to the use of violence as a means of dealing with any frustrating situation they encounter were mostly exposed to violence as victims or as bystanders when they were growing up.

Exposure to evil ideology or culture are some of the pathways through which people get addicted to violence of anger as a way of life. Be very careful the things you allow children to read or watch, especially as cartoons before they imbibe evil ideologies of karma, the survival of the fittest, an eye for an eye, white and black witch etc.

Engaging in activities which are abominable before God

Another secret of addiction which is not directly caused by demons but result as part of the wages of sin is when we do things described by the God of the Old Testament as abominations. Engaging in incestuous sexual relations; engaging in idol worship; consulting with demonic spirits or mediums, having a lying tongue, having wicked imaginations, sowing discord amongst brethren and maltreating the weak in society.

These seven abominations before a righteous God creates a major pathway for the many addictions which plagues societies today. These addictions then bring the consequences that religious people are familiar with such as curses, afflictions, death and poverty.

Proverbs 6:16-19 King James Version (KJV)

16 These six things doth the Lord hate: yea, seven are an abomination unto him: 17 A proud look, a lying tongue, and hands that shed innocent blood, 18 An heart that deviseth wicked imaginations, feet that be swift in running to mischief, 19 A false witness that speaketh lies, and he that soweth discord among brethren.

Keeping our lives free from these things the Lord hates will remove many pathways to addictions from our lives. It will remove many destructive habits which are destroying our suitability for relationships and jobs. It will remove many curses we keep incurring because we are involved in these seven evil practices. Repenting and forsaking such habits will show that we are indeed vessels unto honour and not unto dishonour in the household of Jehovah.

PRAYER NUGGETS

Pathways to Addictions

1) Using substances to assuage or relieve you of negative emotions can lead to addictions.

2) Using demonic substances like charms, books, music and food dedicated to demons can lead to addictions.

3) Partaking in abominable sexual acts, and consulting the fetish or mediums can lead to addictions.

4) Using drugs to overcome fear or using other performance enhancing drugs can lead to addictions.

SECTION III: SIGNS AND SYMPTOMS OF ADDICTIONS

CHAPTER 9

SIGNS AND SYMPTONS OF ADDICTIONS

Signs and symptoms

Signs of addiction show in the addict's observable changed behaviour however symptoms of addiction are the effects the chemical he or she is addicted to produces in the body. Thus signs are observed by a by stander but symptoms are experienced by the addict. When people are addicted they become financially unpredictable, having large amounts of cash at times but no money at all at other times.

The addict will redraw large amounts of money to engage in his or her addiction till he or she runs out of money. The addict will suddenly change his social group often making new and unusual friends and may engage in odd phone conversations at odd times with these new friends.

Another sign addict show is repeated, unexplained outings, often with a sense of urgency. You may also see drug paraphernalia such as unusual pipes, cigarette papers, small weighing scales, etc. at a place he or she frequents or stays.

You may also discover "Stashes" of drugs, often in small plastic, paper or foil packages in the person's things or room. The person will show increasing 'tolerance', thus the need to engage in the addictive behaviour more and more to get the desired effect. Withdrawal happens when the person does not take the substance or engage in the activity, and they experience unpleasant symptoms, which are often the opposite of the effects of the addictive behaviour.

There are seven (7) main signs & symptoms of addictions based on Behaviour, Mood and Changes in the Body.

Unusual Changes in Mood and Body

The addict begins to have extreme mood changes – happy, sad, excited, anxious, etc. He or she may suddenly experience weight loss or weight gain and or unexpected and persistent coughs or sniffles. Though the addict may be originally a healthy person, he or she may suddenly seem unwell at certain times and better at other times for no plausible reason.

Pupils of the eyes seeming smaller or larger than usual in the addict. Bloodshot or glazed eyes can also be a sign of addiction.

Compulsive Behaviours

Difficulty cutting down or controlling the addictive behaviour. The person's life will increasingly be about the addiction and how to support it. Social, occupational or recreational activities becoming more focused on the addiction, and important social and occupational roles being jeopardized.

The person becoming preoccupied with the addiction, spending a lot of time on planning, engaging in, and recovering from the addictive behaviour. Sometimes they are unable to sit still.

Development of Deviant Behaviours

Secretiveness: the person suddenly abandons his or her once outgoing and opened personality and starts hiding things from parents, friends, spouse etc. A once honest person, the addict will start telling lies to get money or space to feed the addiction.

If the substance he or she is addicted to is expensive then the addict may resort to stealing or other criminal activities.

Sudden Mental Illness

Sudden show of mental illness, where there is none in the family. The person may suddenly become violent in deeds or words. The addict may stop taking care of his or her personal grooming and may start dressing very seductively. Though a quiet person he or she may suddenly become a talkative or vice versa.

The once conservative person may suddenly start going out with random people who may not even be found in his or her circles of friends before the addiction. He or she will spend more time with other known addicts.

Abusive Tendencies

Addictions are often triggered by frustrations in life. It is therefore not surprising that many people involved in high pressure jobs deal with the pressure with one addiction or the other. It is therefore common to see addicts displaying sudden abusive behaviours to spouse or children. A mother may neglect to feed children or pay attention when they call for help.

A father may beat an erring child mercilessly instead of using the rod of correction to gently correct him or her. A wife may suddenly become verbally abusive whilst a husband may become physically abusive because of the addiction.

Lack of Interest in Progressive Activities

The addict will start sleeping a lot more or less than usual, or at different times of the day or night than he or she is known for. The addict may show symptoms such as changes in energy: unexpectedly getting extremely tired or energetic for no reason. The once excellent student will come home and claim he or she is no longer interested in schooling without giving any tangible reason. The once vibrant worker will suddenly lose interest in performing his or her duties

Depression

The once vibrant, easy going person will suddenly become reclusive and may fall into depression. Sometime the depression is so severe that they can stare into the void for hours. They may eat so much or very little because of the depression. They may even become suicidal if not helped in time. If it is a chemical addiction they may overdose at this stage because of increasing tolerance of the chemical making it difficult for it to lift them out of their state of moodiness.

The signs and symptoms of addiction can also be classified into three main forms: Physical, Behavioural and Emotional signs and Symptoms of addictions.

Physical Signs and Symptoms of Addiction

Addict exhibits repetitive speech patterns, excessive sniffing and runny nose (not attributable to a cold), looking pale or undernourished and the clothes do not fit as before. An addict may change his or her eating habits and have unusual odours or body odour due to lack of personal hygiene.

Behavioural Signs of Addiction

The addict will start missing work/school work and begin to have problems at school with teachers etc. Addicts may start missing important engagements, isolating themselves from the family. They may isolate themselves and start showing disrupted sleep patterns. Their addiction may start giving them legal and relationship problems.

They may start to have financial problems (e.g. always needing money), a situation which has no logical cause. Their conversations or Google searches may be dominated by using of drugs or drug/alcohol related topics.

Emotional Signs of Addiction

Addicts often become irritable/argumentative, defensive and unable to deal with stress. They may lose interest in activities that used to be part of their lives and become obnoxious, silly, confused and can easily be in denial of the things happening around them. Addicts will rationalize – offering alibis, excuses, justifications, or other explanations for their usual behaviour. Addicts like to minimise: admitting superficially to the problem but not admitting to the seriousness or full scope of the behaviour or consequences. Blaming: addicts will place the blame for their behaviour on someone else or some event but not on themselves. Diversion: addicts change the subject to avoid discussing the topics which concern their addiction.

PRAYER NUGGETS

Pathways to Addiction

1) Signs of addictions show in the addicts changed behaviour however symptoms of addictions show in the changes produced by the substances in the addict's body.

2) There are seven (7) main signs & symptoms of addictions based on Behaviour, Mood Swings and Changes in the Body.

3) The signs and symptoms of addiction can also be classified into three main forms: Physical, Behavioural and Emotional signs and symptoms of addictions.

4) There are about four behavioural changes which show people have become addicts: compulsive behaviour, mental illness, abusive behaviours and deviant behaviours.

SECTION IV: TREATING ADDICTIONS

CHAPTER 10

DEALING WITH DEMON INDUCED ADDICTIONS

Luke 15:17-24 King James Version (KJV)

17 And when he came to himself, he said, How many hired servants of my fathers have bread enough and to spare, and I perish with hunger! 18 I will arise and go to my father, and will say unto him, Father, I have sinned against heaven, and before thee, 19 And am no more worthy to be called thy son: make me as one of thy hired servants.20 And he arose, and came to his father. But when he was yet a great way off, his father saw him, and had compassion, and ran, and fell on his neck, and kissed him.21 And the son said unto him, Father, I have sinned against heaven, and in thy sight, and am no more worthy to be called thy son. 22 But the father said to his servants, Bring forth the best robe, and put it on him; and put a ring on his hand, and shoes on his feet: 23 And bring hither the fatted calf, and kill it; and let us eat, and be merry: 24 For this my son was dead, and is alive again; he was lost, and is found. And they began to be merry.

Surrendering To the Lordship of Jesus

Many people who have been afflicted with addictions by demons are set free when they give their lives to Christ and become born again. The born again experience makes everything new and the spirit of God who comes to leave in the individual then displaces the spirit of the devil. When you become born again your dead spirit as an unbeliever is raised back to life unto righteousness. The born again spirit will then expel whatever demons where residing in the individual at the place meant for his spirit. If those spirit were responsible for addictions in his or her life then that addiction goes with them.

Rededicating Your Life to Jesus

There are people who fell into sin as Christians and continued in the sin till they moved from being controlled by their born again spirit to being controlled by their flesh. The once born again Christian at this stage is called a backslidden Christian. Such a person has a mental knowledge of righteousness but has no conviction to carry it out. Such a person has now become accustomed to listening to the doctrines of demons. Such a person has by now lost the ability to discern between his spirit and that of demons. But like the prodigal son above he should come to his senses because of the pains of the addiction so he will be given a second chance by the father in heaven. Many once vibrant Christians are now addicts who now eat in the spirit with pigs or demons, food not meant for children of God. Who now indulge in acts that sometimes shock unbelievers because they are now under the influence of demonic spirits. The beginning of relief for the addict or backslidden Christian is the admission that I have sinned against my father in heaven and therefore needs to go back to him and submit to his wishes. And be ready to do whatever he asks no matter how demeaning.

In verse 19 he said '*And am no more worthy to be called thy son: make me as one of thy hired servants.*' He was ready to have no rights and even ready to do hard work without commendation or praise. He was ready to have no opinion but to follow without question what the father instructed. In this mind-set of a servant he demolished the four major obstacles of deliverance from addictions: 1) thinking you are special; 2) having a strong opinion; 3) stubbornness and 4) unwillingness to work hard without praise. After the backslidden Christian has rededicated his or her life to Christ, he needs to be taken through a deliverance sections to restore his ability to discern between the voice of the Holy Spirit and that of the devil or his agents. After the deliverance section the restored backslidden addict needs to be counselled to form a new mind-set to resist the edge to get back to the addiction. Having a servant mentality in following the father in heaven by following the instructions of the Holy Spirit will demolish any addiction and its urges in the life of the man or woman who has rededicated his or her life to Christ.

Expelling the Demonic Strongman

Mark 5:1-5 King James Version (KJV)

1 And they came over unto the other side of the sea, into the country of the Gadarenes. 2 And when he was come out of the ship, immediately there met him out of the tombs a man with an unclean spirit, 3 Who had his dwelling among the tombs; and no man could bind him, no, not with chains: 4 Because that he had been often bound with fetters and chains, and the chains had been plucked asunder by him, and the fetters broken in pieces: neither could any man tame him.5 And always, night and day, he was in the mountains, and in the tombs, crying, and cutting himself with stones.

Dealing with the gateway demon or the controlling demon in the life of an addict is crucial. The demon who made room for all the other demons to come in: the demon acting as landlord of your body and leasing it out to other demons to strengthen the addiction. Like Legion who made the mad man of Gadara addicted to pain: the Bible says he screamed all the time, lived in the cemetery, cut himself with stones and went about in the cold and rainy days naked. This man to the outside word was having a mental problem but it was actually a demonic problem caused by one demon opening the door for several thousand demons to get into his host. The strongman needs to be discerned and the sin or behaviour which serves as a gate or entry pass for it to enter the body destroyed so he does not come back with more demons to create a worse situation than originally existed in the possessed after deliverance.

Asking for the baptism of the Holy Spirit

Acts 1:8 King James Version (KJV)

8 But ye shall receive power, after that the Holy Ghost is come upon you: and ye shall be witnesses unto me both in Jerusalem, and in all Judaea, and in Samaria, and unto the uttermost part of the earth.

The Holy Spirit is the third person of the Godhead and therefore has all power. Under the Old Testament men who had the Holy Spirit on them where men of renowned. Men of incredible strength, unchallenged wisdom, great vision bearers. The Holy

Spirit also endowed women with great administrative skills. The power of the Holy Ghost transformed errand boys into kings, timid people into warriors who were able to liberate nations and even gave David the ability to transform impoverished people in Israel into mighty men of valour.

The baptism of the Holy Ghost makes tremendous power available unto the believer. But for the Holy Ghost, the message of the gospel would not have turned the world upside down without armies or swords. The power of the gospel is essentially the power of the Holy Ghost. The baptism of the Holy Spirit which is the overflowing of the Holy Spirit in a Christian with its initial sign of speaking in tongues empowers the Christian to fight addiction. Praying in tongues on a regular basis therefore strengthens the Christian to deal with any behavioural, emotional or even desire induced addictions that may be bothering him or her. The fruit of the spirit is therefore the outcome of the process of the Holy spirit working on the heart, mind and body to overcome tendencies to yield to lust which leads to addictions.

Galatians 5:22 King James Version (KJV)

22 But the fruit of the Spirit is love, joy, peace, longsuffering, gentleness, goodness, faith,

The fruit of the Spirit is only exhibited by people who are no longer under the bondage of addiction. Because addicts are certainly not joyful, peaceful, gentle, faithful nor patient when it comes to getting another fix.

PRAYER NUGGETS

Dealing with Demon Induced Addictions

1) The backslidden who have demon induced addictions get relieved when they rededicate their lives to Christ.

2) Unbelievers with demonic addictions or afflictions are often set free when they surrender their lives to Jesus Christ.

3) The baptism of the Holy Spirit also produces enough power to drive out addictions.

4) Dealing with the gateway demon or the controlling demon in the life of an addict is crucial for setting him or her free from the addiction.

CHAPTER 11

TREATING SUBSTANCE ADDICTION

Holy Ghost Substitution

The Bible says that we should not be drank with wine wherein there is excess but be drank with the Holy Ghost. We dealt extensively with the power of the Holy Ghost to deal or remedy addictions in the preceding chapter.

Ephesians 5:18 King James Version (KJV)

18 And be not drunk with wine, wherein is excess; but be filled with the Spirit;

The scripture above is teaching the fundamental truth which runs through all addictions, excess. A substance addiction is simply a dependence on a drug, nicotine or alcohol to a point where it is used in excess. Paul is saying that the best way to remedy our substance addictions is to be filled with Holy Ghost. The word filled in the scripture above means to be complete or to be filled to the brim. To be so supplied with the spirit that any addition leads to overflowing. Many born again, Holy Ghost filled

Christians will tell of the many substances they were addicted to but were able to overcome after the baptism of the Holy Spirit. These miracles took place because the emotional inadequacies which drove people to the addictions or kept them addicted were dealt with in a genuine born again experience. The feeling of emptiness which many try to feed with drugs or nicotine is then filled with the Holy Spirit who brings joy unspeakable in a new believer.

Come Give your life to Christ and You can Smoke all You Want

I once read a story which illustrates the truth of salvation in its ability to deliver people from addictions without any other therapy. Once a lady went to one of the old American evangelist and told him she had heard the message he preached but she needed time to quit her smoking habit before she could come to the alter to give her life to Christ. The evangelist then told her to come just as she is because the gospel is for sinners and not saints.

Then to this addict's shock he added, come and give your life to Christ and if you feel like smoking you can go back to it and smoke all you want. Thinking she could still eat her cake and have it she quickly run to the altar to surrender her life to Jesus. After she had become born again the crusade run for a number of days. One of the days the evangelist run into this nicotine addict and asked her about her addictions since she gave her life to Christ. She happily told him that she had lost the taste for nicotine after she surrendered her life to Christ and has since not been able to smoke.

This is why there is an Akan proverb which says that it is unwise to stand in the middle of soldier ants whilst trying to prevent them from climbing your body to bite you. No one can be in an environment or emotional mode which feeds an addiction whilst still trying to remedy that addiction. To deal with addiction friends involve in the addiction will need to change, the environment of the addict which supports the habit needs to change and the habit of consuming the substance causing the addictions needs to change too.

Like the medical therapies used in rehabilitation centres the addicts will have to be put on substitution therapy. They will have to be given substituted substances which gives similar experiences like the drugs or nicotine they are addicted to but are not themselves addictive. The best substitute for the Christian addict is hours spent each day praying in tongues.

Prayer

Prayer is indeed the master key and by engaging God in this way you can access help from above to pull through any addiction you might be going through. Repenting of the emotions or desires which led to the addiction in prayer is a very good foundation for recovery. Then presenting the need to overcome your addiction before your father in heaven after confessing and forsaking your sinful ways is a very good next step towards recovery. The Bible says that we are more than conquerors through him: indeed we have more power than the power of a conquering army. More power than a conquering army behind an emperor of old because the creator of the universe is on our side.

Romans 8:37 King James Verse

37 Nay, in all these things we are more than conquerors through him that loved us.

Again the Bible says that God has empowered us such that we can do all thing through Christ who strengthens us. These 'all things' certainly includes regaining control over our own bodies and minds which has been taken over by drugs, nicotine or alcohol addiction.

Philippians 4:13 King James Version (KJV)

13 I can do all things through Christ which strengtheneth me.

Deliverances

Luke 15:17-24 King James Version (KJV17 And when he came to himself, he said, How many hired servants of my father's have bread enough and to spare, and I perish with hunger! 18 I will arise and go to my father, and will say unto him, Father, I have sinned against heaven, and before thee, 19 And am no more worthy to be called thy son: make me as one of thy hired servants.20 And he arose, and came to his father. But when he was yet a great way off, his father saw him, and had compassion, and ran, and fell on his neck, and kissed him.21 And the son said unto him, Father, I have sinned against heaven, and in thy sight, and am no more worthy to be called thy son. 22 But the father said to his servants, Bring forth the best robe, and put it on him; and put a ring on his hand, and shoes on his feet: 23 And bring hither the fatted calf, and kill it; and let us eat, and be merry: 24 For this my son was dead, and is alive again; he was lost, and is found. And they began to be merry.

The story above has been told many times to illustrate the need for those who are not born again to stop their rebellious ways and return to the father in heaven. But a careful look at this story will also tell of an addict who wasted his inheritance on his addictions. The Bible says that it was after 'he came to himself' that he realised he was in bondage and decided to free himself by going back to the father, to submit to him as his son. This means he did all the wasteful spending because he was addicted to shopping, sex, alcohol and the desire to waste resources.

He so wasted his inheritance to a point where he was left penniless and in great need. He still tried to hold on to the addiction by scrapping for it with odd jobs till he sank as low as to share with pigs. Before he saw the delivering hand of God in his life and then decided to return to the environment which will support his addiction free lifestyle, his father's house.

Procrastination

Procrastination has always been seen to be a very bad habit or tendency. Procrastination has the following signs and characteristics which prove that it is a bad habit: Chronic lateness, Poor time management, Putting off tasks, Difficulty meeting deadlines, Difficulty making decisions, Difficulty prioritizing and accomplishing tasks, Making excuses and distracting from completing important tasks. I have come to realise that procrastination can be put to some good use.

Procrastination, I believe, is the most effective way to stop a bad habit. From my own experience it is the best way to undo something that has been done for so long that it now happens automatically. I believe procrastination's sole positive purpose is to render ineffective the process which keep repeating an addictive behaviour. Procrastinations makes the process which leads to needing a fix or the process which leads to momentary pleasure from an addictive substance or behaviour ineffective.

Procrastination destroys the ability to reach goals by introducing lateness, putting of tasks, missing meeting deadlines and failing to accomplish tasks. Applying these characteristics of procrastinations to your addiction will make its occurrence difficult and its controlling power over the addict ineffective. Procrastination is so powerful that it has rendered resource rich nation poor because leadership keep postponing the tackling of difficult but necessary decisions.

I get uncomfortable when people compare Ghana with South Korea when talking about how far the later has gone economically ahead of the former. They make this comparison of a country which is now a developed country to it lower middle income counterpart because they got their independence around the same year and had similar economic indicators. They do not however add that at some point in their history the leadership of

South Korea tasked its people to surrender their jewellery to rescue their economy. They never mention that the people of South Korea work so hard that most of their economically active citizens, due to the pressure of work are addicted to alcohol. None of the sacrifices the citizens of South Korea had to make to grow their economy has been demanded of the people of Ghana. Neither did Ghana get the kind of support South Korea got from the United States to fight the Communist North. The defining difference between the two nations is the leadership they have both had in their over sixty years after independence.

One leadership encouraged citizens to give their all to build their nation whilst the other's leadership's incompetence led to the citizens giving less and less of themselves for the building of their nation over the years. Even as you may begin to experience withdrawal symptoms as you keep postponing your fix from minutes to hour and to days. You will need to pray for strength to endure, it is the brain throwing tantrums because it is losing control of your mind and body.

Here, alcohol is an essential part of daily life for many, with South Koreans drinking more hard liquor than anyone else in the world, according to the research firm Euromonitor. It is cheap, considered a must if you want to get ahead in business and viewed as a way to relieve stress in a society with some of the *world's longest working hours. But South Korea is also home to more alcoholics than any other country, and alcohol-related social costs amount to more than $20bn a year, Ministry of Health and Welfare estimates show* (Chao, S & Gooch L., 2018).

PRAYER NUGGETS

Treating Substance Addictions

1) Using procrastination as a strategy to delay acting out the addictive behaviour till the compulsions to yield wanes enough for you to regain control of your actions.

2) Replacing the need to be 'high' with the power of the Holy Ghost where in there is no excess.

3) There is also the process of taking the addict through a deliverance session where the power of the substance he or she is addicted is broken to bring about total relief.

4) Praying for strength to deal with the withdrawal symptoms of not taking the substance you are addicted to will bring the inner strength to pull through till the addict regains his or her mental strength to say no and mean it.

CHAPTER 12

BEHAVIUORAL ADDICTIONS

Introduction

Every behaviour we exhibits was learned at one point or the other in our lives. Because it had a beginning it can also be ended. Every actions we take produces responses which encourage us to repeat or stop them. Our character is a composite of our habits, which we have been allowed to repeat so often that we no longer need consciousness to execute them. Our character is simply a reflection of our dominant behaviours. What is the significance of this truth? It is significant because when someone has a bad character he or she blames it on nature and not nurture. Why is this a potent excuse? If it is nature then there is nothing he or she can do to change it. But if it is nurture then he or she had made it and can therefore unmake it. The responsibility to change a bad behaviour is put right on his or her door step. The need for a change will then drive him to make amends.

Humans are born with the tendency to be foolish and need corrections from parents or guardians so that foolish behaviour is discouraged but proper behaviour is encouraged. A child who is not weaned of foolish behaviour grows up with it and becomes a behavioural addict of one sort or the other. If the unpleasant action of using a rod is not sustained the child will grow up thinking there is no painful consequence to foolish behaviour.

Proverbs 22:15 King James Version (KJV)

15 Foolishness is bound in the heart of a child; but the rod of correction shall drive it far from him.

In the same way an addict will have to make up his or her mind to suffer the pain of undoing behaviours which have brought good feelings over many years because of its negative consequences.

Meditation on the Word

Meditation on the word of God helps because the world is active and powerful and sharper than any two edged sword. Meditation on the word is concentration on a particular portion of scripture by repeating it in the mind continually till the word comes alive in your heart. In this state the Christian empties himself or herself of all the distractions of the world to focus on the word of God.

Because the word of God is active and alive it will begin to grow in the heart and set to work freeing the addict from the entanglement of his or her addiction. The word has power to divide the spirit and the soul of a man. As the word grows in the heart it will cut the addiction chains that bind it. The word will then begin to produce ideas which are contrary to the ideas produced by the substances or behaviour causing the addiction. As the word grows in the mind it will overcome the ideas or imagination produced by the addiction till the addict breaks free.

The word indeed has power to go deep into our blood cells and can permeate into the bones of an addict. Meditate on the word till it comes alive in your heart .It will serves as the sieve of your thoughts and intentions and help control what enters your thoughts. Addictions are strongholds because they are designed to be self-sustaining.

Hebrews 4:12 King James Version (KJV)

12 For the word of God is quick, and powerful, and sharper than any two edged sword, piercing even to the dividing asunder of soul and spirit, and of the joints and marrow, and is a discerner of the thoughts and intents of the heart.

But like any stronghold its weakest link are the people already within it. Because its heaviest fortification are without whilst its protection within is usually weaker. Discerning through meditation on the word therefore turns the 'people' or thoughts in this case within the stronghold against it. Once the addict's thoughts are full of the word of God it will fight the evil imaginations which often instigate and fuel the addiction. No addictions can persist without evil imaginations.

Evil imaginations are the gateway for any addictions. Without evil imaginations there is no real pleasure in addictions to keep it going. Substance abuse is so difficult to treat because it produces its own imaginations called hallucinations. These imaginations then give this false sense of bravado, happiness, tranquillity, thrill and invincibility to the addict even as they are destroyed.

Deliverance from Behavioural Addictions

Sometimes the addict has gone so far as to undo what he or she is doing by himself or herself through sheer mental strength. If he or she is has become possessed by demons because of a continuous sinful lifestyles or the addict is under the oppression of demonic spirits then deliverance from the spirit of addiction will be needed. There are many people walking around with addictions because in church there is the belief that a Christian does not need deliverance. Yes a victorious Christian does not need deliverance but one who has backslidden because he or she is living in sin certainly does. Bible says we will have to rescue people from the very fire of hell. Why will someone need rescuing if the person is not in bondage? From time to time leadership of churches need to call for people with addictions to come for prayer. They need to pray that church members are not led to addictions by the choices and imaginations they encounter daily. Most backslidden Christians who do not repent will end up in hell because of their sinful addictions. Addictions are the number one cause of hypocrisy in church. People are ashamed of what they do in secret but are too afraid to open up for fear of being looked down upon after it becomes public.

Procrastination as a Strategy to Deal with Behavioural Addictions

Every behavioural addiction starts in the mind and is entrenched by repeated action till it gains a live of its own. As someone who has personally had behavioural addictions, I am more than sure that procrastinations as a strategy is able to neutralise its hold on the individual. Most addictions are done in secret but behavioural addiction often show up in public much to the embarrassment of the addict. I believe you were shocked to hear of certain actions by people you held in high esteem in society. You might have heard of the scandal for the first time but they might be addictions plaguing them for years but no one knew. Behavioural addictions usually affect those who are close to the addict because they cause sicknesses, pain and loss.

Dealing With the Root Desire or Craving Feeding the Habit

Every behaviour of human beings is aimed at fulfilling a desire. Hence man's obsession with how he feels at all times since it could predict his past, present or future actions. A man acts because he feels or desires: that is the way of all men who are not led completely by the Holy Spirit. Deal with the desires or feelings sustaining the addiction by building up your born again spirit through tongue speaking.

Once the feeling or desires subsides the motivation to continue in the addictive behaviour to fulfil that feeling will also diminished, giving the addict the opportunity to form better behaviours to counter the addictive ones. Hence the ability of a born again spirit to change a person who was once addicted to a sinful lifestyle into a model citizen of his or her community. The most effective way to mortify the flesh with its desires is through regular periods of Bible study accompanied by prayer with fasting.

PRAYER NUGGETS

Behavioural Addictions

1) Dealing with the root desire or feeling feeding the habit will eventually stifle the addiction because it will be out of fuel.

2) Behavioural addictions are habits which are out of control because they are inspired by a feeling or desire that is out of control but the process can be truncated when procrastinations is to yield to the addiction is employed by the addict.

3) Procrastinations can also be an addiction that plagues individuals or even nations. I believe the only positive use of it is to undo bad habits and addictions.

4) Meditations on the ever active and powerful word of God gradually rewrites the evil code written in the heart and mind feeding addictions which destroy the lives of addicts.

CHAPTER 13

DESIRE RELATED ADDICTIONS

Deliverance Ministration

The desire for love recognition, fame, fortune and power are some of the strongest drivers, pushing people into many habits which become addictions. There are people who drink alcohol excessively because of the desire to be free of stress, abuse and marginalisation. Others are driven to addictions of over eating or starvation because of the desire to be appreciated or admired. These addictions if instigated by demons can all be dealt with through deliverance from an anointed servant of God. Once the demon inducing that addiction is driven out the addict then regains the strength to decide what to do with his or her life.

Non Stop Reading or Listening to Anointed Messages

There is power in the word of God, hence the need to listen or read it constantly. There is power in it because it is by the same word that the worlds were made by the Lord. The Bible says that:

you have been set free because of the word you have heard even the word of grace. We have learnt that imaginations and desires are the chief fuels for any addiction. These fuels get their source from the things we hear and especially from the ones we pay attention to. Controlling what we hear, desire or imagine. Consistently listening to the word of God will drive away demonic influences and keep out thoughts centred on the things which build us up spiritually.

Dealing with the reasons for the desire.

Desires are only symptoms of actions we strongly want to take place or judgement of events which have already taken place. Desires can also arise in anticipation of an event or in response to touch, sight or words. Desires can also be stirred by the things you encounter or hear because they can be cravings, a yearning or aspiration. Best of all, desires are a product of the soul, a language expressing our opinion of things which affect as or the things we care about. There are people whose addictions can be traced to fear, sadness, depression, anger or loneliness. These are the commonest feelings or desires which feed most addictions. These feelings are either caught through upbringing or taught by religious or local leadership.

There are whole nations or religions whose members have similar reactions to the same issues because of the same yearnings or aspirations they share though they may live in different countries. A careful enquiry into the life of the addict or through revelation by the Holy Spirit can identify the root cause of the desire which is feeding the addiction. Once the root cause is identified and dealt with, the addictions ceases to have a foundation to stand on and can through prayer and counselling be remedied. People who feel unloved or unwanted fall into many addictions as they seek for love. Similarly people with low self-esteem are also prone to many forms of addictions as they adopt all kinds of habits to please the crowd which accepts them.

PRAYER NUGGETS

Dealing with Desire Related Addictions

1) Dealing with the reasons for the desires causing the addictions through prayer and counselling till the addict is free.

2) Non Stop reading or listening to anointed messages creates the atmosphere which drives away demonic influence which destroys the foundation of addictions.

3) The frustrations of people who could not fulfilling their desires or aspirations have led many to do drugs to cope with the shame and disappointment they feel.

4) Deliverance Ministration helps the addict who has been afflicted by demons with the power to be free of that addiction.

CHAPTER 14

DEALING WITH RELATIONSHIP RELATED ADDICTIONS

Renouncing the relationship

Philippians 4:13 King James Version (KJV)

13 I can do all things through Christ which strengtheneth me.

All across the globe there are women and men who are in very abusive relationships but will swear they are having the time of their lives despite the cuts, bruises and broken bones. Many have being murdered young because they could not get out of relationships with wicked men or women. Their addictions to the momentary pleasure the relationship brought from time to time made weaning themselves of their abusive partners nearly impossible. But in Christ any Christian can do all things including weaning himself or herself from a relationship that he or she is invested in materially or emotionally.

Every relationship begins with an agreement. There is always an offer by one of the parties and an acceptance by the other. On the basis of that a covenant is created within which the relationship then functions. It does not matter what name they call themselves so long as they are emotionally and or sexually invested in each other, the union is spiritually recognised and needs a higher spiritual power to annul it. The Bible confirms this by saying that: no two people can walk together excerpt they are agreed.

Amos 3:3 King James Version (KJV)

3 Can two walk together, except they be agreed?

Disagreeing with the person's behaviour does not annul the relationship but a proclamation that you no longer want the relationship and want nothing to do with him or her because he or she has broken his or her promise to respect and honour you will do it. Then you repent of any evil you might have been involved in and ask for restoration from the Lord. Lastly you need to move from the person's sphere of influence till your emotions are under your control once more.

Deliverance Ministrations

There are lustful spirits which help keep backslidden Christians bound in sinful and abusive relationships. Others are addicted to relationships because they get entangled in soul ties because of the type of covenants they enter into at the beginning of their relationships. Some innocent people at the height of their love emotions are driven to fantastic proclamations to their relationship partners. Some even partake in blood covenants which subsequently open them up to demonic afflictions or possession. People under the influence of demons are often afflicted with uncontrollable desires and made to feel their emotional needs are not being fulfilled. Such people often lack self-control when it comes to the man or woman they love. With the mighty hand of God such demon induced addictions are set aside during deliverance sessions and the addict is immediately relieved of his or her urges.

Many backslidden Christians who have developed addictions need to rededicate their lives to the son of God who is able to save them once again. Any addict who allows the son of God to stay in his or her life will be set free completely by his power. Released to contract relationships which glorify God and uplift the image of every child of God who is in love.

John 8:35-36 King James Version (KJV)

35 And the servant abideth not in the house for ever: but the Son abideth ever. 36 If the Son therefore shall make you free, ye shall be free indeed.

Dealing with the reason for dependence on that Relationship

1 Corinthians 6:12 King James Version (KJV)

12 All things are lawful unto me, but all things are not expedient: all things are lawful for me, but I will not be brought under the power of any.

When basic needs like love, security, recognition and acceptance are not met people often result to using the desires of the flesh to fill the vacuum created. The pleasure derived from habits which produce 'the feel good effect' or the 'feel good hormone induced feelings' work for a while and then begin to wane because the underlining need has still not been met. Then more has to be done with even more intensity to produce the same pleasure the addict has grown used to.

Subsequently what seems like the 'solution' becomes another problem that if not checked, spills out of control. It is in this (i.e. cycle of need met with a wrong solutions which creates even more needs), that the wisdom in the scripture above becomes clearer. Do not engage in a habits for the sake of having short bouts of intense pleasure or that emotion will grow to a master which will control your very life. If you have a relationship, emotional or social need, then connect with the people concern and be frank about it. Being open will release the pent up feelings which can grow to an obsession which will later drive you to excess. This pent up feeling from childhood can push you to love the wrong gender or even believe you are trapped in the wrong body. Being open about what is bothering you in life is the first step towards dealing with secrets which feed addictive behaviours in relationships.

PRAYER NUGGETS

Dealing with Relationship Related Addictions

1) Renouncing the relationship which are abominations before God and praying for his strength to walk away from it will do you a lot of good.

2) If it was an abominable relationship then most likely demons will be involved. For the addict to be free therefore he or she need to go through deliverance.

3) Deal with the reason for the dependence whether it is fear of loneliness or of poverty and the dependence will have no foundation to stand on.

4) You cannot stop something you agree to no matter how much you complain. To stop a relationship you do not like therefore, confess in prayer your desire for it to end and the lord will empower you to do so even as you sever contacts with the person till you are free of his or her influence.

SECTIONS V: WHEN ADDICTIONS ARE NOT TREATED

CHAPTER 15

EFFECTS OF UNTREATED ADDICTIONS

Madness

Many people addicted to drugs, both prescriptions and hard drugs, if they continue in that addiction unabated will keep losing control of their minds and inhibitions till they finally lose their minds altogether. In Ghana, most young men who lose their minds is as a result of addiction to marijuana or some other hard drug and for the young women it is mostly as a result of issues with heart break.

Demonic Possession

People involved in sexual or emotional addictions over a long period become exposed to demonic possession or oppression. There are people who are addicted to emotions like anger, sadness and so on. As the person lends herself to continuous self-pity or temper tantrums it opens the person up to demonic possession if an unbeliever and demonic oppression if a backslidden Christian.

Death

Almost daily people overdose drugs like cocaine in the western world after years of addiction to that drug. This situation has happened to both addicts who are poor and to those who are rich with the ability to access the best medical care. Addiction to sadness which is often called depression has led many to seek death as the only way out of it.

Renders Individuals Unproductive

Go to any ghetto or poor neighbourhoods in the developed or developing world and you will see young men and women who because of addictions have become a burden to their nations. People who have become too occupied with their addictions to be good for any productive venture. A man who after several attempts by his mother to rehabilitate him of drug addiction was eventually cut out her will. He lost his present and future wealth which would have come out of his inheritance to addiction.

Brings Poverty

There are people who have sold all they have just to feed an addiction. I know of a renowned musician who squandered all his millions on addiction to cocaine till his former bands mate had to give him money to feed. He died still very poor compared to his mates who were not addicts despite his incredible talent of playing the organ. Addictions have rendered generations upon generation in certain families poor and wretched. Womanizing, doing of drugs, alcoholism, gambling, wasteful expenditures and addictions like that have made families, societies and even nations wallow in poverty.

Leads to Divorce

I cannot count the number of men who lose their marriages because of alcoholism. Men who spent most of their pay check just bringing shame to their families as they spend their nights in the street or gutters because they are drunk. People addicted to gambling have gambled the fortunes of their families away, leading to the wife or husband leaving the marriage.

Leads to Chronic Diseases

I know of a colleague worker who was addicted to very hard liquor. The heavy drinking day in and out over the years caused the cirrhosis of his liver. The doctor warned him to stop drinking or lose his life but he still could not and ended up dying as predicted. Sexual addictions have led to sexually transmitted diseases which have killed millions over the years.

Abusive relationships

Very good husbands or wives have suddenly become physical or verbally abusive because their addictions have made them loose control of their actions. Indeed people who become addicted emotionally to a woman or man outside the marriage become abusive caring no longer about their spouses or even children. I know of a man who because of addiction to a woman picked his children under the pretext of taking them on holiday and dumped them on their maternal grandmother.

This man forgot his own children because of an emotional addiction to another woman with her own kids. This man fed his own children with the same food every day for months whilst feeding another man's children with sumptuous meals because of his feelings for their mother. Check any abusive relationship and you will notice there is an addiction of one or more kind of the spouses.

Many people try advising people involved in such relationships to no avail, forgetting that their behaviour has gone beyond habit to an addiction. They are trapped in that cycle of destructive behaviour and need rescuing before they can act sensibly or responsibly.

PRAYER NUGGETS

Effects of untreated addictions

1) Abusive relationships are sometime caused by the unreasonable behaviour of an addicted partner or spouse.

2) Addiction leads to a lot of waste of resources to keep the expensive habits going. But result in unreasonable behaviours which mostly leads to job loss culminating into the poverty of the addict.

3) Renders Individuals Unproductive in their endeavours in business or as employees because it makes them neglect their duties.

4) Addictions to sinful lifestyles and the continuous practise of evil behaviours due to addictions can lead to demonic possession.

SECTION VI: MAINTAINING YOUR DELIVERANCE FROM ADDICTION

CHAPTER 16

STAYING FREE FROM ADDICTIONS:

- **1) Living in righteousness**
  The devil is coming but he has nothing with me a famous statement by Jesus to his disciple. Living in righteousness which is not by law but by grace is the surest way to stay away from any addiction. For the righteous is as bold as a young lion to say no to all the evil temptations that come his or her way.

  John 14:30 King James Version (KJV)
  30 Hereafter I will not talk much with you: for the prince of this world cometh, and hath nothing in me.

- **2) Avoiding Lustful images and films**
  I have made a covenant with my eyes that I will not look at a woman lustfully. Job was able to stick to one wife despite all the temptations he might have faced as a very rich man. Do not patronise lustful movies, books or songs and your mind will be kept from impure thoughts.

  Job 31:1 New International Version (NIV)
  31 I made a covenant with my eyes not to look lustfully at a young woman.

- **3) Learning to forgive**
  The Lord forgives us our trespasses as we forgive those who trespass against us. In forgiveness a lot of rage and painful desires to retaliate is lost leaving the individual free of any emotional burdens. By harbouring these feelings and desires a vacuum is created in the individual which eventually sucks him or her into addictions. Emotional and behaviour addictions which can lead the offended doing worse things than the one who offended him or her.

  Matthew 6:14 New International Version (NIV)
  14 For if you forgive other people when they sin against you, your heavenly Father will also forgive you.

  Mark 11:25 King James Version (NIV)
  25 And when you stand praying, if you hold anything against anyone, forgive them, so that your Father in heaven may forgive you your sins."

- **4) Memorising scripture**
  Your word have I kept in my heart so I will not sin against you is true because the word produces faith which lead to righteous decisions. Not knowing the word or ignorance of the word leads to faithlessness which deny us the promises of God. The word in the heart fight against addictive tendencies.

  Hosea 4:6 King James Version (KJV)

  6 My people are destroyed for lack of knowledge: because thou hast rejected knowledge, I will also reject thee, that thou shalt be no priest to me: seeing thou hast

forgotten the law of thy God, I will also forget thy children.
Psalm 119:11 King James Version (KJV)
11 Thy word have I hid in mine heart, that I might not sin against thee.

- **5) Developing the Habit of praying in tongues**
He who prays in tongues edifies himself and lifts his spirit above the flesh. At this stage his righteous spirit is able to exercise better control of his body by overcoming the temptations which lead to addictions.

  1 Corinthians 14:4 King James Version (KJV)
  4 He that speaketh in an unknown tongue edifieth himself; but he that prophesieth edifieth the church.

- **6) Accepting Counselling from Godly men and women**
In a multitude of counsellors is safety. There is an adage which says: you cannot be too careful in life. That it is better to err on the side of caution than without it. Surround yourself with wise people and you will be wise.

  Proverbs 11:14 King James Version (KJV)
  14 Where no counsel is, the people fall: but in the multitude of counsellors there is safety.

  Proverbs 15:22 King James Version (KJV)
  22 Without counsel purposes are disappointed: but in the multitude of counsellors they are established.
  Proverbs 24:6 King James Version (KJV)
  6 For by wise counsel thou shalt make thy war: and in multitude of counsellors there is safety.

- **7) Learning to be quick to confess and forsake sins**
  If I hid iniquity in my heart the lord will not hear me. Harbouring of evil thoughts and ideas in the heart is the fuel which keeps addictions raging.

  Psalm 66:18 King James Version (KJV)
  18 If I regard iniquity in my heart, the Lord will not hear me:

- **8) Learning to be humble**
  Pride goes before a fall but he who humbles himself shall be exalted. Humility is needed to submit to the discipline needed to overcome addictions and to stay of it for good.

  Proverbs 16:18 King James Version (KJV)
  18 Pride goeth before destruction, and an haughty spirit before a fall.

- **8) Developing The Habit Of Waiting On God**
  They that wait upon the lord shall renew their strength and shall mount up with wings as eagles.

  Isaiah 40:31 King James Version (KJV)
  31 But they that wait upon the Lord shall renew their strength; they shall mount up with wings as eagles; they shall run, and not be weary; and they shall walk, and not faint.

- **9) Developing Self-Control**
  Self-control is the discipline that makes you deny yourself of something you deserve or have access now because

of a better reward in the future. I will develop self-control to keep in check my desires and feelings so as to avert addictions.

Galatians 5:22-23 New International Version (NIV)
22 But the fruit of the Spirit is love, joy, peace, forbearance, kindness, goodness, faithfulness, 23 gentleness and self-control.

DECISION PAGE

If you are not born again the promises in this book cannot be your portion because they are meant for those redeemed by the Lamb of God who takes away the sins of the world. If after reading this book you want to be born again say these words aloud wherever you are right now and Jesus will come and live in your heart.

Dear Lord Jesus forgive me for all my sins against you and cleanse me with your precious blood shed on the cross of Calvary. I forsake all my past evil deeds and plead that you take me and make me part of the family of God. Remove from me any curse that is following me because of my bloodline and link me to the blessings of the children of Abraham. I promise to obey and follow you all the days of my life. Please baptise me with the Holy Spirit and with power for the Christian walk.

Amen.

If you prayed the prayer above aloud then Congratulations! You are now a born again Christian and a child of God. If you are not in any church find a well-established church which believes in the baptism of the Holy Spirit with the evidence of speaking in tongues and commit to it with all your strength, gifts and talents.

Please write to me and tell me how this book has impacted your life to the following addresses

C/O TIDD/Forestry Commission

Box 783

Takoradi

Western Region, Ghana

Email Address: lexgyi@yahoo.com or lexgyi@gmail.com

OTHER BOOKS BY THE AUTHOR

1) Fear versus Faith: The Battle for the Control of Your Destiny.

2) 5 Things I Wish I Had Mastered By Age 30 For A Life Of Excellence.

3) 20 Things I Wish I Had Mastered By Age 30 For A Life Of Excellence.

4) But: Key for Turning Sinking Sand Into Stepping Stones.

5) Familiarity and the Anointing.

6) His Great Grace Breaks Barriers.

7) Talents: Treasures In Earthen Vessels.

8) 15 Things I Wish I Had Mastered By Age 30 For A Life of Excellence.

BIBLIOGRAPHY

1) https://jamesclear.com/new-habit: How Long Does it Actually Take to Form a New Habit? (Backed by Science).Copyright © 2018.

2) Jump up ^ "mind – definition of mind in English | Oxford Dictionaries". Oxford Dictionaries | English. Retrieved 2017-05-08.

3) www.merriam-webster.com/dictionary/stronghold © 2018 Merriam-Webster, Incorporated.

4) American Society for Addiction Medicine (2012). "Definition of Addiction".

5) Dictionary.com Unabridged. Based on the Random House Unabridged Dictionary, © Random House, Inc. 2018

6) www.drugs.com/slideshow/prescription-drug-addiction-1075#Prescription Drug Addiction: Top Facts for You & Your Family. Medically reviewed on Mar 28, 2018 by L. Anderson, PharmD.

7) Collins English Dictionary – Complete and Unabridged, 12th Edition 2014 © HarperCollins Publishers 1991, 1994, 1998, 2000, 2003, 2006, 2007, 2009, 2011, 2014.

8) American Heritage® Dictionary of the English Language, Fifth Edition. Copyright © 2016 by Houghton Mifflin Harcourt Publishing Company. Published by Houghton Mifflin Harcourt Publishing Company. All rights reserved.

9) Bressert, S. (2017). Histrionic Personality Disorder. Psych Central. Retrieved on November 19, 2018, from

https://psychcentral.com/disorders/histrionic-personality-disorder.

10) 8 Common Behavioural Addictions. Everyday Health© 1996-2018 Ziff Davis, LLC. Everyday Health is among the federally registered trademarks of Ziff Davis, LLC. Retrieved on November 22, 2018.

11) Windle, L. (2017) The Sun. Living Teen's plastic surgery to look like Angelina Jolie goes very wrong. November 17, 2017, 3:58pm.Chao, S & Gooch L. (2018),The country with the world's worst drink problem. Al Jazeera Media Network.

www.ingramcontent.com/pod-product-compliance
Lightning Source LLC
Chambersburg PA
CBHW031233250726
48655CB00005B/1935